AVOIDIN … ER
ONE DAY AT A TIME

PRACTICAL ADVICE FOR PREVENTING CANCER

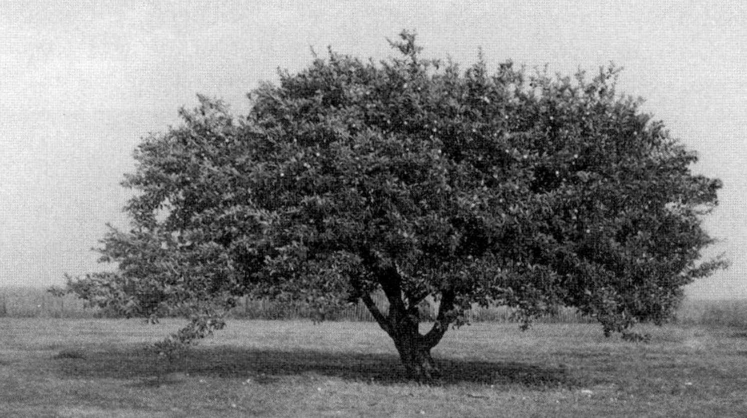

LYNNE STOESZ-ELDRIDGE, M.D.
DAVID BORGESON, MS, MPT

Beaver's Pond Press
Edina Minnesota

DISCLAIMER: The information presented in this book is not a substitute for proper medical care. It is designed to augment information about cancer prevention that you obtain from regular medical check-ups and screenings.

This information is based on research and is aimed at preventing and not treating cancers. If you have been diagnosed with cancer, consult a medical provider before observing the nutritional and lifestyle approaches presented here. Some of the nutrients that show promise in helping to prevent cancer could actually render cancer treatment, such as chemotherapy, less effective.

The evidence presented about chemicals that may cause or prevent cancer is imperfect. Studies are being conducted which will provide further information in the next few decades. We will be thrilled if some of the possible carcinogens we list turn out to be completely safe in twenty years.

These practical pointers may not prevent you from getting cancer. It is our hope that they will suggest ways you can raise the odds in your favor.

All of the examples used as illustrations in this book are fictional or composites of many experiences we've had with patients. Any circumstances that resemble those of our readers are purely coincidental.

Illustrations by Rachel Wick and Russell Eldridge

ISBN-13: 978-1-59298-159-5
ISBN-10: 1-59298-159-3

Library of Congress Catalog Number: 2006909633
Printed in the United States of America
First Printing: November 2006

10 09 08 07 06 5 4 3 2 1

Beaver's Pond Press, Inc.

7104 Ohms Lane, Suite 216
Edina, MN 55439
(952) 829-8818
www.BeaversPondPress.com

To order, visit www.BookHouseFulfillment.com, or www.avoidcancernow.com
or call 1-800-901-3480. Reseller discounts available.

To: Joy 1/1/11

DEDICATED

to

Peter,

Philip,

Timothy,

David,

Jennifer

and

Jessica

Love,

Lori

Table of Contents

"The Doctor of the future will give no medicine,
but will interest his patients in the care of the human frame,
in diet, and in the cause and prevention of disease."

—Thomas Edison

Acknowledgements

Writing this book would not have been possible without the help of many people to whom we are deeply indebted. To our patients, family, and friends with cancer, we offer heartfelt thanks for allowing us to participate in your lives and, through your experience, to "catch" the passion to prevent these dreaded diseases.

I (Lynne) wish to thank my children and family for their patience with my research, and for being "subjected" to a cancer-prevention lifestyle. I also thank all of you for your humor, as you in turn "subject" others around you to these principles!

I (David) wish to thank my wife, Beth, for her support and patience, and my sister, Lynne, whose persistence and confidence in me kept me on track.

Many others have provided countless hours of support and, though nameless here, we want to express how truly grateful we are for your help. We express thanks to Jennifer Manion, our editor, not only for her many helpful suggestions, but for sharing our passion to prevent cancer. To Lynette Schultz, friend and literary guru, we send praises, for her almost instantaneous ability to see the big picture. We also wish to thank Milton Adams of Beavers Pond Press for his guidance and experience in navigating us through the process of publishing this work.

Finally, we wish to express utmost thanks to David Wick for his steadfast patience, exceptional planning and organization, and breath of encouragement that brought this book to life. We love you dearly.

INTRODUCTION

"I keep the subject of my inquiry constantly before me, and wait till the first dawning opens gradually, by little and little, into a full and clear light."

—Isaac Newton

This book is the culmination of an effort by the authors to reduce some of the heartache we have seen repeatedly in our patients, friends, and family stricken with cancer. While some cancers are the result of risky behaviors, too often this villain attacks young, otherwise healthy people, even children who are going through life minding their own business. They have heeded warnings that we might compare to tornado or hurricane warnings, but the warnings have been incomplete or have come too late. Unless we are certain disaster will strike, we are often afraid to appear over-reactionary and go out on a limb. This book is written for those who are seeking something before the sirens blow.

We have watched friends develop cancer at young ages. We have witnessed friends become widowed with young children. We have grieved the agony that cancer pain has inflicted on our older friends and relatives. None of these people were abusing their bodies. None of them smoked, drank to excess, or lived on hot dogs. Yet with 80-95 percent of cancers having an environmental component, perhaps something could have been done differently to "save" their lives before their cancers started.

This book is about **primary** prevention. This is defined as preventing something **before** it actually begins. The National Cancer Institute defines primary prevention as:

1. Avoiding a carcinogen or altering its metabolism.
2. Pursuing lifestyle or dietary practices that modify cancer-causing factors or genetic predispositions.

There is a third category involving medical interventions to treat preneoplastic (precancerous) lesions. With the exception of dietary measures that may hasten the clearance of cancer causing viruses, these interventions lie outside the scope of this book.

Secondary prevention is the art of searching for cancer once it has started and finding it before it spreads out of control. Early detection has its merits, has been written about extensively, and is practiced daily in primary care clinics. Examples of secondary prevention include recommendations about when to do self-breast exams or have a screening colonoscopy. Chapter Ten contains current recommendations for secondary prevention based on the American Cancer Society's recommendations. Screening that extends beyond these basic recommendations may be considered for those with a family history of cancer.

Tertiary prevention is beyond the scope of this book and includes methods to support an individual after they are diagnosed with cancer. Some of the information presented here may play a role in tertiary prevention. The treatments for several cancers predispose individuals to other cancers and advice here may apply in that setting. The authors recommend carefully discussing your diet with your oncologist if you have been diagnosed with cancer. Some of the nutrients and phytochemicals discussed could actually work against treatments for cancer.

This book is designed to provide practical and, in many cases, simple ideas to decrease your risk of developing cancer. We believe that a fanatical, obsessive approach to preventing cancer is not necessary. Frequently, a commonsense, moderate stance is the most beneficial. It is our belief that being healthy should be FUN and we have attempted to make the chapters on prevention an interesting launch pad to start you thinking, not a boring text to be followed sleepily.

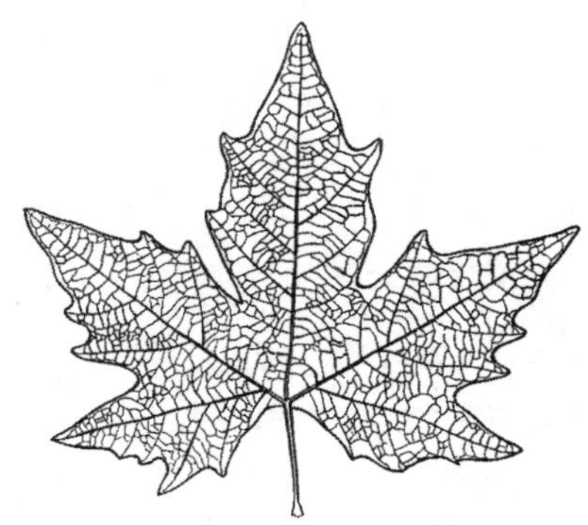

Chapter One

What Are We Doing to Prevent Cancer?

"Economics and politics simply intertwine in shaping conventional medicine's approach to cancer. Very simply put, treating disease is enormously profitable, preventing disease is not."

—The British Cancer Control Society

Why, despite the billions of dollars spent on research to find a cure, have we failed to make a dent in the overall mortality from cancer for over sixty years? Although the age-adjusted death rate from 1950 until now has halved for heart disease and pneumonia and nearly quartered for strokes, it has not budged for cancer. The reason is not because we are living longer. This is what "age adjusted" means in this statement. It would be easy to cast the evil eye at tobacco, but smoking during this time in the U.S. decreased from nearly 50 percent of adults to less than 25 percent. The incidence of cancer has risen steadily; however, in 2006 in the United States, it appears the incidence may be declining slightly. Unfortunately, the same experts who celebrate this exceptionally modest decline are not hopeful it will continue as the baby boom generation hits peak cancer time. According to the World Health Organization (WHO), global cancer rates could increase by 50 percent to 15 million by 2020. One out of every two American men and one out of every three American women will get cancer over the course of their lifetimes.

There are many foundations such as the American Cancer Society and the Leukemia and Lymphoma Society dedicated to finding cures. Significant advances have been made in the treatment and survival rates for a few types of cancer, such as childhood leukemia and Hodgkin's disease. Despite this, the five year survival rate for cancers overall has not changed significantly since 1950. Only about 50 percent of people diagnosed with cancer live longer than five years.

So what are we doing wrong? Why has the mortality from heart disease dropped dramatically, while that from cancer has remained essentially unchanged?

We believe a significant factor is that our society is driven by money, and that far more money is allocated to treating rather than preventing cancer. There is great potential for financial gain in developing and marketing an effective chemotherapy agent. There is little financial incentive in preventing the tumor the drug would treat. There is clear financial incentive in treating animals and crops with hormones, pesticides, and antibiotics in order to raise production and increase crop yield. There is little financial reward in evaluating what these substances do to our bodies once we ingest them.

Perhaps we physicians should bear a burden to teach, yet we live in a managed-care society that increasingly requires physicians to see more patients with less financial reward. Insurance companies reimburse physicians to spend an hour counseling a patient about how to proceed after a cancer is diagnosed. There is little or no reimbursement for educating patients about how to prevent that cancer, or, for that matter, any cancer, in the first place.

As physicians, we are also limited by a lack of knowledge. I (Lynne) recall many lectures in medical school dealing with the diagnosis, etiology (cause), and treatment of various cancers, and spending many hours looking through a microscope discovering the differences between normal and malignant (cancerous) cells. I do not recall a single lecture on cancer prevention. I also recall many lectures discussing the biochemistry of proteins, carbohydrates, and fats, and studying the mechanisms by which vitamins work in our bodies. I recall only one lecture on clinical nutrition meant to apply this knowledge to practice.

We as consumers are also at fault. We want cheaper food. We want convenience. We do not want to go to the store daily, so we want foods with a long shelf lives and, hence, preservatives. We are willing to spend thousands of dollars and explore alternative medical practices once we are diagnosed with a tumor, but we spend little to educate ourselves about ways of avoiding disease in the first place. Part of the problem is the magical thinking that we accuse our teens of having: it will be someone else, especially someone who is not as health-conscious, who will get sick. Yet of the 80-95 percent of cancers that have an environmental component, only one third are due to smoking.

Governmental agencies have limited funding and are not the answer. Despite anti-smoking campaigns, anyone over the age of eighteen can freely buy carcinogens at the corner store, and we have even spent our hard-earned dollars subsidizing the tobacco industry.

At least for now it is up to us as individuals to educate ourselves and adopt lifestyles consistent with cancer prevention. Physicians do not have the time to educate patients sufficiently. The government is unable to protect us completely. The pharmaceutical companies are going to invest more of their resources into drugs rather than the prevention of something the drugs would treat, and this is to be expected. We would not expect the automotive industry to invest more money into developing methods of eliminating cars than in manufacturing them! Food manufacturers will continue to find methods of increasing supplies to respond to the consumer's demand for cheaper, longer-lasting food.

We can no longer be complacent and expect our best interests to be looked after by others. It is up to us to take charge of our own bodies and lives!

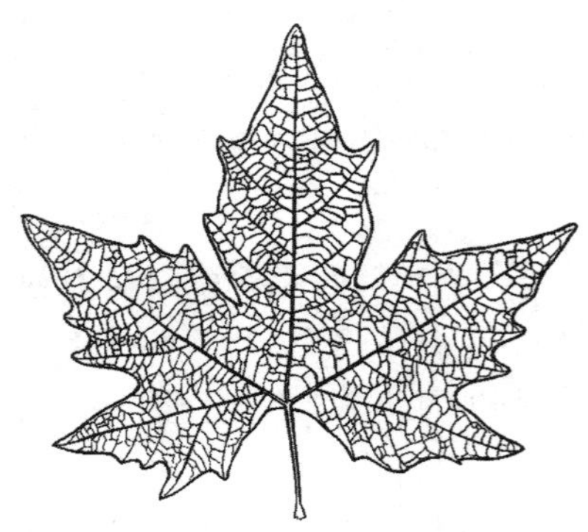

Chapter Two

Cancer Prevention IQ Pretest

"Prevention is better than cure."

—Desiderius Gerhard Erasmus

(Answer yes or no to the following questions; if a question does not apply to you, answer yes)

1. *Have you had your home tested for radon, knowing that radon is the second leading cause of lung cancer in the United States and that excess levels are found in one out of fifteen homes?* no

2. *Do you sleep in total darkness?* yes

3. *Do you have houseplants in your home that NASA has found effective in absorbing formaldehyde, benzene, and trichloroethylene emissions?* yes

4. *Do you exercise at least thirty minutes daily?* yes

5. *Do you drink green tea?* no

6. *Do you know which foods tend to contain pesticide residues, and hence should be ingested only if grown organically?* no

7. *Is your body mass index twenty five or lower? (If you are uncertain what this is, see the table on page 96)* yes

8. *If you have well water, have you had it tested?* no

9. *Do you eat at least five servings of fruits and vegetables daily?* no

10. *Do you avoid antibiotics unless they are clearly needed for a bacterial infection?* yes

11. *Do you avoid establishments where smoking is allowed?* yes

12. *Are you aware of which viruses, bacteria and parasites predispose a person to developing cancer?* no

13. *If in a monogamous relationship, do you have a healthy sex life?* yes

14. *Do you have access to a list of known carcinogens to help you evaluate the safety of household products?* no

15. *Are you up to date on cancer screening procedures that are recommended for you, based on your age and sex?* yes

16. *If you purchase decaffeinated beverages, do you make sure they are decaffeinated by the Swiss method or another non-chemical method?* no

17. *Do you avoid dry-cleaning, and either wash your clothes or take them to a "wet" cleaner?* yes

18. *Have you made a detailed medical family history chart for yourself and shared this with your physician?* yes

19. *If your children play on outdoor, wooden playground equipment, do they always wash their hands and take showers or baths after playing?* n/a

20. *Do you practice safe sex?* yes

21. *Do you use primarily stainless steel, glass, and ceramic in cooking, and throw away any non-stick cookware if it shows any damage?* yes

22. *If you have a history of gastritis or peptic ulcers, have you been tested for* ***H. pylori*** *bacteria?* n/a

23. *Do you avoid foods high in acrylamide such as french fries?* yes

24. *Do you have an active spiritual life?* yes

25. *Do you choose dietary supplements carefully and only with the help of a knowledgeable professional?* yes

Answer Key:

If you answered "yes" to 23 to 25 of the questions, excellent. You could have written this book. Keep up the good work.

If you answered "yes" to 15 to 23 questions, very good. You are motivated; paying attention to a few points in this book could raise your odds of avoiding cancer even further.

If you answered "yes" to 10 to 15 questions, good. Read this book carefully. You have a good start and we hope to provide you with many pointers to help you live a long cancer-free life.

If you answered "yes" to 2 to 10 questions, you have a lot to learn. It is never too late to apply principles outlined in this book. Even small changes could change your life.

If you answered "yes" to 0 to 2 questions, don't despair! It is never too late to adopt preventative measures!

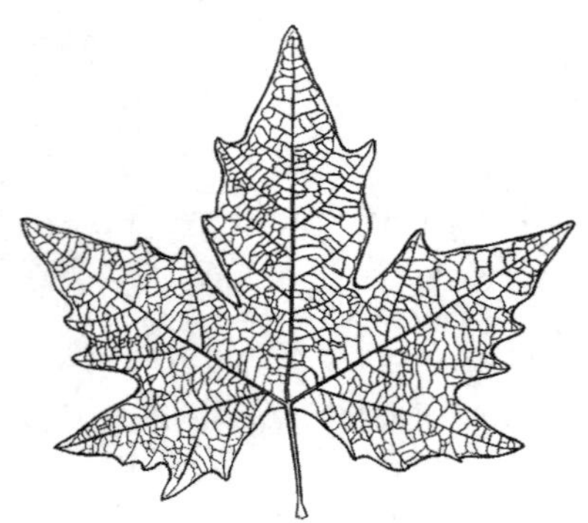

Chapter Three

What Is Cancer and What Causes It?

"Growth for the sake of growth is the ideology of the cancer cell."

—Edward Abbey

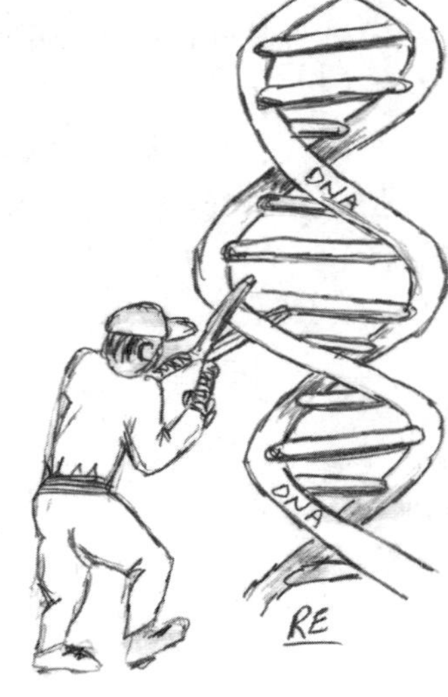

Paper Jam

Cast:

Mr. Antiox	Antioxidants
General Practitioner	Family doctor
Geek ONC SWAT Team	Oncologist
Radical Groups	Free radicals

Office Your Body

DNA Inc computer	DNA/genetic code
Embedded hard drive errors	Genetic mutations predisposing to cancer
Hard drive errors	Acquired DNA mutations
Low crime rate area	Non-smokers
Intermingled outlet cords	Invasive cancer
Grenades and poisons	Chemotherapy

ACT ONE

Scene One:

Your office was running smoothly. From personnel to office supplies, no expense had been spared in the start-up. Your state of the art computer system made by DNA Inc. appeared infallible. Sure, there were a few small errors embedded in the hard drive, but this was common. In an age where free roaming radical groups loomed everywhere, you chose a location where the crime rate was relatively low. Of course, your office was still vandalized by some of these radicals, as all offices are, but your office manager, Mr. Antiox and his team were prepared. Together they held a defense that foiled most attempts the radicals devised to shut down DNA Inc. The several small hits DNA took were difficult to quantify but did not seem to affect the systems operations. Incident reports were filed, but life went on.

Scene Two:

After many successful years in operation, you begin to question whether your office is working with the efficiency at which it did before. Production is down; the supply cabinet is running low, and you are going through ink and paper faster than ever before. Being an astute businessperson, you quickly call upon the building caretaker, General Practitioner to evaluate the situation. The General checks out your office and finds that a mass of papers have been building up behind the printer. He also finds that the printer is no longer communicating with DNA Inc. Worse yet, he is unable to turn it off manually since the cords to the outlet have intermingled with the cords to vital office systems.

Scene Three:

Papers begin to overwhelm your shredder as the General makes a call to the printer SWAT team, Geek ONC. Although brilliant, the technicians do not have the ability to log on and switch off the printer. Since, they know so much more than when you purchased your first computer ages ago, they inform you that there are several errors on your hard drive resulting from daily wear and tear and the vandalism. Because of this, DNA Inc is no longer able to control the printer. They even have a very good idea where these errors lie. They know what needs to be done, if only they could get there…

Scene Four:

Limited by their current technology, the Geek Onc. SWAT team rounds up the weapons they have. With their laser guns, grenades, and poisons they launch an all out war on the printer. As the printer slows down, you breathe a wavering sigh, as you see that the attack has caused extensive office damage as well. Further attacks compromise the office more than the printer has, and the mission is called off. You burst into tears, knowing this office was your life, and there is nothing you can do to save it from the printer. The printer SWAT team steps back sadly, and the printer drains all remaining energy from the office, effectively pulling its own plug.

Act Two

Scene One:

You wake up trembling; you are sweating from every pore. You pinch yourself more than once to make sure it was a dream. As you make your way to the kitchen for a glass of water, you write yourself a note to meet with your office manager, Mr. Antiox, in the morning to increase the surveillance around your office.

Fade scene...

Cancer is a group of more than 100 diseases that begin in a single cell, defined by the type of cell or body system involved. A cell can change from normal to cancerous following an accumulation of several mutations. Some of these mutations are inherited and account for the genetic predisposition to some cancers. Most mutations are acquired after birth. Of these, some happen spontaneously as an error in the normal reproduction of cells.* The likelihood of these mutations rises with anything that causes cells to reproduce more often, such as repair of inflammation. Some mutations are due to direct DNA damage from free radicals generated by normal bodily functions or by environmental insults. Even if a cell suffers a handful or two of mutations, most of these cells self-destruct or are scavenged by the immune system.

*Considering each of our trillion cells contain our genetic code of DNA, which in turn consists of 3 billion "letters" that must be duplicated accurately each time a cell divides, it seems remarkable to the authors that cancer is not more common.

The term "tumor" can refer to both benign and malignant growths. Benign (non-cancerous) tumors can grow quite large at times, but do not spread (metastasize) to distant sites. They are, in general, more of a nuisance than a danger unless they occur in an enclosed space such as the brain. Examples of benign tumors include lipomas (fatty lumps commonly found below the skin throughout the body) and ovarian cysts. Malignant tumors, or cancers, are distinguished by the course they take. Cancers can spread (metastasize) to distant sites.

Causes of Cancers

There are many "causes" of cancers, a number of which will be discussed at greater length in later chapters. The important point to keep in mind is that one food does not prevent, and one chemical alone does not necessarily cause, cancer. Despite the fact that cigarette smoking clearly causes lung cancer, the incidence of lung cancer is lower in Japan where there is also a greater percentage of smokers.

But Why?

Cancer is a multifactorial disease. Simply put, several elements combine to either produce or eliminate a cancer cell. We are all exposed to carcinogens daily, yet we do not all develop cancer.

Again...why?

Studies of immigrants demonstrate that factors other than genetics play a large role in the development of cancer. Japanese women have a low incidence of breast cancer. If they move to Hawaii, their risk increases, and it increases further if they move to the mainland United States. It is clear that genetics alone cannot explain this, and such studies strongly suggest an environmental role in the development of cancer.

Timing is also critical. Times of rapid growth, for example, during pregnancy, where the babies' cells are multiplying rapidly and differentiating (changing into different tissue types), are different than times of slower growth seen in an adult.

During these rapid growth periods, the body is more susceptible to environmental insults. If DES (a hormone) is given to a one-month-old mouse and the administration continues through its lifetime, no effect is noted. If, however, DES is given to a pregnant mouse, the offspring are predisposed to developing cancer. It is well known that infections such as German measles (Rubella) and cytomegalovirus (CMV) cause only mild illness in children, but can be devastating to and cause multiple defects in a child born to a woman who contracts these while pregnant. Likewise, a small dose of a chemical at a critical time during pregnancy can have a greater effect and cause more mutations than the same chemical introduced at another time in life.

Studies to evaluate whether a substance causes cancer are, in general, done on healthy, young male subjects. It is unknown what an acceptable level of exposure to most carcinogens would be for a pregnant woman, young child, or adolescent going through puberty, and these studies, for ethical reasons, will probably never be done

Distribution of Causes of Cancers—An Overview

I. GENETIC
5-20 percent of cancer deaths are due to inherited mutations

II. ENVIRONMENTAL (non-genetic) 80–95 percent of all cancer deaths, including 5-15 percent due to an inherited mutation combined with environment

Tobacco—25-40 percent of all cancer deaths

One third of all cancer deaths and almost 90 percent of deaths from lung cancer are due to smoking.

Diet and obesity—25-30 percent of all cancer deaths

Obesity, or being overweight, alone accounts for 14 percent of cancer deaths in men and 20 percent of cancer deaths in women in the United States. According to the International Agency for Research on Cancer (IARC), as many as 375,000 cases of cancer could be prevented each year in the U.S. through healthy dietary choices. In a person of normal weight, dietary changes can also play a significant role in decreasing the risk of cancer and are discussed in detail in chapters Six and Eight.

Infection—10-25 percent of all cancer deaths

In the United States, it is estimated that around 10 percent of cancer deaths are related to infection, whereas infections cause 25 percent of cases worldwide. The leading culprits in the U.S. include human immunodeficiency virus (HIV), giving rise to multiple cancers, human papillomavirus (HPV); which causes cervical, anal, vaginal, penile, and oral cancers, hepatitis B; associated with liver cancer, hepatitis C; associated with liver cancer and lymphomas, and H. pylori; associated with stomach cancer.

Ionizing/UV Radiation—2-7 percent of all cancer deaths.

UV radiation causes 90 percent of skin cancers. Radon is the second leading cause of lung cancer.

Occupational—2-8 percent of all cancer deaths

Exposure to occupational hazards accounts for around 5 percent (6-10 percent in men and 1 percent in women) of cancer deaths, especially those involving cancers of the lung, bladder, and bone marrow.

Pollution and environmental chemicals—less than 1 to 5 percent of all cancer deaths

In the United States, chemicals and pollutants account for roughly 1 to 5 percent of cancers. In other regions of the world, for example Chernobyl, Ukraine, pollution accounts for a much higher percentage of cancer.

Physical inactivity—1–2 percent of cancer deaths

Regular physical activity is associated with a decreased risk of developing breast and colon cancers, probably decreases the risk of developing prostate cancer, and may lower the risk of developing lung and uterine cancers as well.

Alcohol—3 percent of cancer deaths

Alcohol has been shown to have a causal link with the development of cancers of the breast, liver, mouth, esophagus, pharynx, larynx, colon, and rectum. Alcohol currently is currently felt to be responsible for 3.6 percent of all cancers; 5.2 percent of cancers in men, and 1.7 percent of cancers in women.

STUDIES ON CANCER CAUSES

"It has recently been shown that research causes cancer in rats."

—Author unknown

To understand how researchers determine if something causes or possibly causes cancer, and the limitations researchers face, it is necessary to have some understanding about cancer studies. Many of the studies conducted to evaluate substances for the ability to cause cancer are done on animals. In these studies, the animals are frequently given very large doses of the suspect substance. This is done to maximize the chance of detecting even a small risk, and to determine if there is cause for concern within the constraints of the study time. Many studies are conducted over a period of weeks to a few years. Most substances that are known to cause cancer require exposure over a period much greater than this, a time frame known as a latency period. This is the period of time between exposure to the offending substance and detection of cancer. With most cancers, the latency period is at least fifteen to twenty years. This is the reason for the jokes the authors have heard over the years. Why should I be concerned about such and such if I do not eat forty-seven pounds of it daily as the rats did in the study?

Since it is unethical to give people 47 pounds of a possible carcinogen to see if it causes cancer, studies on humans are designed to compare groups of people without cancer (called a control group), to a similar group of people with cancer. Retrospective studies are designed to look back in time comparing the two groups, looking for differences in things such as environmental exposures or dietary habits. Prospective studies are designed to look forward in time and are in general more accurate since variables are controlled at the outset. These studies can be helpful if a substance or environmental hazard with a short latency period (something that takes only a few years to cause or prevent cancer) is being studied. For a prospective study to demonstrate a cancer risk from a substance with a long latency period after exposure, however, would require a study designed with results not obtainable for several decades. Many of these studies are currently in progress.

Weighing the Risks

"Life is a risk."

—Diane Von Furstenberg

A few thoughts to contemplate before reading on: In the following chapters, the authors present information in order to bring awareness to the public about possible cancer dangers, as well as about a few cancer-fighting treasures they may not be aware are sitting in their refrigerators. We cannot emphasize enough the importance of maintaining perspective when delving into the dos and don'ts of cancer prevention. Our hope is to provide information to help people enjoy a healthy life and lifestyle and have fun. If we observe someone chain smoking or numbing their mind with martinis because his or her children had nitrate-laden hot dogs for lunch, our point will be lost. If we witness our readers embracing a few points but perhaps disregarding others, our goal will be achieved. This goal is to present basic facts (or what is currently known) based on solid scientific studies about an area ridden with conflicting reports and hype. The Internet is a remarkable asset, but is laden with "false-truths" as well. Can you really get cancer from wearing pink toenail polish during a full moon if you sleep on the wrong side of the bed?

People tend to make judgments about risk based more on fear than on facts. The thought of an asteroid on a course anywhere near earth heightens our senses more than do the thousands of drunk drivers on inebriated courses down the roads we are driving. "Genetically modified food" raises a proverbial red flag, while our national flag remains folded in a closet next to multiple chemicals that may cause cancer. The author's have experienced these judgments firsthand through our love of hiking. The facts tell us that we are more at risk during our travels from a motor vehicle accident, being struck by lightning, or even being stung by a bee. Fear tells us that a grizzly bear is waiting around the next corner. We take precautions based on our fear, and hike in groups, carry bear bells, and watch the trails for bear droppings. Based on facts, we should perhaps make it a higher priority to avoid driving at dusk, take cover at the first stroke of thunder, and stay clear of beehives.

There is tremendous controversy over what causes and prevents various cancers, and much of the research is preliminary and incomplete. In the next several chapters, we have evaluated many studies looking at possible causes of cancer. In many instances, there are studies that show an increase in cancer in one case, while the next study shows no increase. Our goal is not to determine whether the studies are conclusive beyond any doubt. It is to introduce the reader to substances that have either been shown to elevate or decrease cancer risk in reliable, well-thought-out studies.

This book is not meant to produce fanatics, but to help health-conscious people achieve healthier lifestyles with respect to cancer prevention. Many substances that appear to be protective against cancer when taken in moderation (such as calcium and dairy products) may increase the risk of cancer when taken in high amounts. If your child is dehydrated and the only rehydration solution available contains a food dye, do not become overly alarmed. A small exposure in this case may very well be warranted in order to prevent more serious issues and illness. Have either of the authors ever stood outside while pumping gas, consumed more than the recommended limit of trans fats per day, or treated themselves to products containing the preservative BHT? The answer is an overwhelming yes. Moderation and a general awareness of concerns in our environment are key.

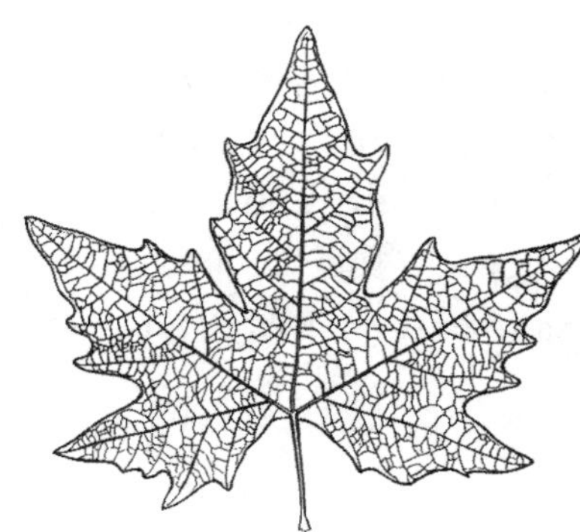

Chapter Four

The Environment And Cancer Prevention

"Concern for man himself and his fate must always be the chief interest of all technical endeavors...in order that the creations of our mind shall be a blessing and not a curse to mankind."

—Albert Einstein

It took thirty years and thirty million dollars to prove a causal relationship between smoking and cancer. This presents an uneasy thought, since studies to evaluate cancer risks from particular substances show that the more widespread the use, the more likely an association with cancer will be detected. This is if the substance or chemical is studied at all. Currently, only two percent of chemicals used in commerce have been tested for carcinogenicity (the ability to cause cancer). Knowing this, should we retreat to the hills, banish all chemicals, and eliminate all technology except that required to build a large bubble around our new community, one meant to screen out the dangers celebrated by our ignorant brothers and sisters?

Before pulling out the washboard and saddling your horse, bear in mind that, of all the environmental carcinogens, the greatest threats to our health have been here all along. Radon and sunlight account for more cases of cancer each year than do the multitude of chemicals we have introduced into our environment in the last sixty years. Certainly we do not want to dismiss possible dangers in our path, and this chapter reviews many such dangers. We simply caution the reader to remember a few of the known dangers while viewing possible concerns, lest while distracted they lose their focus and run off a cliff while looking up at the sky, contemplating a matter that later proves to be trivial.

General Precautions and Personal Protection

"Science is simply common sense at its best."

—Thomas Huxley

Given the products and chemicals we are exposed to on a daily basis—some man-made, some natural, some known to contribute to cancer, many that have not been evaluated—practicing general caution and common sense is our first priority. With infectious disease, we practice universal precautions, safety measures we take to avoid acquiring infections via our skin, eyes, airways, and nasal passages. Applying the same principles to non-infectious, but possibly dangerous substances, could likewise provide protection with little effort. A few simple means of decreasing your exposures follow.

Open Windows and Use Good Ventilation

Indoor air pollution is a significant concern, with indoor air pollutant levels being much higher than outdoor levels. In 1987, the Environmental Protection Agency ruled that, of environmental problems analyzed, indoor air pollution ranked fourth in cancer risk. This has become more of a concern with homes becoming tighter and more energy efficient, allowing pollutants to accumulate. Many common products we bring into our homes release carcinogens, such as formaldehyde, that linger in the air. A tightly sealed home could lower your electric bill, but raise your risk of cancer. Limit indoor use of chemicals and paints to only those chores that must be done indoors, otherwise choose the garage or outside for doing projects. When using such products inside, open as many windows and doors as possible and run exhaust fans. We provide a list of dangerous household products, as well as examples of safer alternatives, later in this chapter.

Gloves

Our skin is not a lead shield protecting us from the elements around us. Many chemicals can be absorbed through the skin. This is more evident now that several medications, including high blood pressure medications, pain medications, hormone replacement therapy and even nicotine, are available in transdermal (patches applied to the skin) therapy. If you would not swallow a product, think twice about allowing it on your skin.

Interestingly, some of the first documented cases of cancer caused by environmental/occupational exposure occurred by the absorption of chemicals through the skin. In 1775, chimney sweeps were found to have significantly elevated rates of scrotal cancer due to exposure to soot that penetrated their pants and their skin. Soot is now a known human carcinogen.

We recommend using impermeable gloves when working with household products and chemicals. Latex allergy is becoming an increasing problem, particularly among those people such as healthcare workers who routinely use gloves. If you note any reaction while wearing these gloves, make sure to switch to the latex-free variety.

Masks

The use of masks can protect your airways from the onslaught of dangerous substances in the environment. It is important, however, to know the correct, effective type of mask to use, lest you think you are avoiding harmful chemicals when you are not. There are three basic types of masks available in many hardware stores. These include inexpensive dust masks that provide some protection from large particles and run around $2.00. The next step up is HEPA filter masks that run from $15.00 to $30.00. These are much better than a simple dust mask if you will be exposed to products such as fiberglass, and they provide more protection against wood dust. The third major type is a fume mask. This type of mask should be used if you will be working with fumes such as in aerosols, solvents, paints, and any pesticides or herbicides. Fume masks usually sell for around $40.00.

Some exposures require much more elaborate filtration, such as the use of respirators. Recommendations for these are usually covered under the material data safety sheets for various chemicals. In these cases, make sure you research the proper mask to use. A proper mask could cost several hundred dollars, and you may want to consider hiring a professional who has been trained in the safe use of the substance.

Leave all products in their original container

If you are unable to read a label on a product, you cannot know if the product in the container contains carcinogens and practice appropriate caution. Transferring products to another container also raises the risk of poisoning, and increases the chance of accidentally combining products such as ammonia and bleach that can react with catastrophic results.

Dispose of hazardous materials safely

Check labels on products you use to see if they can be placed in the normal garbage or if they have special disposal requirements. Items that may require special disposal include unused paint, used motor oil and antifreeze, lead acid batteries (car batteries), fluorescent bulbs, insecticides, and pesticides. Check with your local recycling facility, the city in which you live, or call your garbage service to see where you can dispose of such products. Many cities have adopted annual clean-up days when special disposal service is available as well.

Wash new clothes and bedding items before using them

Clothing and linens that are labeled "permanent press," "wrinkle resistant," or "easy care" are manufactured using a formaldehyde resin, a suspected carcinogen.

Washing these items before using them could remove some of the residual formaldehyde. It is impressive that the authors first learned this tip, and were taught to have an awareness of residual chemicals, by their grandmother who was born in 1909.

Take your shoes off indoors

Removing your shoes when entering your home can reduce your exposure to chemicals such as pesticides, asphalt, and weed-control products that may be present on the bottoms of your shoes and could be tracked through your home. This can also help keep your rugs clean, decreasing the need for chemicals to clean them.

Be aware of toxic chemical releases by industries in your neighborhood

The public has access to information on releases of toxic chemicals to the environment via air, water, and soil by industry. The Environmental Protection Agency's (EPA) Toxic Release Inventory (TRI) contains information from certain industries and federal facilities that are required to submit information about chemical releases to EPA annually. The Web site www.epa.gov/tri has an entry for zip codes so that individuals can access information about chemical releases in their neighborhoods.

Radiation

"Minnesota is ahead of most states in innovative, healthy things like smoking bans, but there are no regulations that make people test for radon or for builders to build radon resistant homes."

—Cecil Keen

Radon

The U.S. Surgeon General has reported that, following smoking, radon is the leading cause of lung cancer in the United States. Radon is a radioactive gas released from the normal decay of uranium in soil and rocks. Radon enters your home through cracks in the foundation, floor, and walls; through openings around sump pumps and drains; and through gaps around pipes and wires. Radon can also be present in the water supply in homes that have well water. The states with the highest risk of radon exposure are North Dakota, Montana, Washington, Pennsylvania, New York, New Jersey, Colorado, and Maryland, but high levels have been found in every state. It is estimated that one out of fifteen homes has a radon level above acceptable levels, defined as 4pCi/L. The average home in the United States has a level of 1.3pCi/L. It was once thought that homes without basements were considered safe, but radon should be checked for in this case as well. Unfortunately, there is no way to predict whether a home will have an abnormal radon level without testing. Levels can vary significantly even among homes in the same neighborhood, and both older and newer homes can pose a risk for radon exposure.

You can have your home tested or purchase a do-it-yourself kit at a retail store. Both short-term and long-term kits are available. If you select a short-term kit it is recommended that you repeat the test in three months. To find out more about test kits, contact the National Safety Council at 1-800-767-7236, the U.S. Environmental Protection Agency (EPA) at 1-800-SOS-RADON, or check out the EPA Web site at www.epa.gov/iaq/radon. You can purchase discounted kits for $9.95 by calling the National Radon Helpline at 1-800-557-2366. Kits should be placed at the lowest level in your home where there is living space.

Radon exposure can be reduced significantly if detected and managed through venting techniques that are not cost prohibitive. The cost of repair usually runs between $800.00 and $2,500.00, a bargain considering approximately 21,000 people in the U. S. die each year because of cancer caused by radon exposure. The National Safety Council operates the National Radon Fix-it-up Program, which is a free service that provides guidance to people whose homes have elevated radon levels. They can be contacted at 1-800-644-6699 and provide support based on the level you obtain through testing. They'll even recommend contractors familiar with repairing radon problems.

If you are looking for a new home, be sure to have the prospective home's radon levels checked. Any problems should be noted in the purchase agreement. If you are selling your home, make sure to check the radon level. Normal levels can be a positive selling point; if levels are not normal, repair the damage prior to selling. If you are building, invest the money in measures that will make sure your home is radon resistant. The savings in the end could be substantial.

Ultraviolet light

Often we fret about hidden environmental pollutants we are exposed to while we worship the sun, one of the most dangerous exposures, and worship it we have, with fervor, up to just a few decades ago. The sun-worshipping days spent perfecting tans in the 60s and 70s have given way to the skin cancer days of the early 21st century. It is estimated that 40 to 50 percent of people who live to the age of sixty five will develop some form of non-melanoma skin cancer over the course of their lifetime. The lifetime risk of malignant melanoma, the "bad" form of skin cancer, is one in eighty four, an increase from only one in 1500 in 1935. Since 90 percent of skin cancers are easily curable, we tend to view these significant numbers somewhat lightheartedly. Yet, for at least 10 percent of those diagnosed with skin cancer, the prognosis is more dismal than one requiring a day off from work and an unsightly scar.

There are three primary types of skin cancer. Non-melanoma skin cancers, which include basal cell carcinoma, and squamous cell carcinoma, tend to grow locally and usually do not spread until they are quite large and noticeable. Of the one million people diagnosed with skin cancer in the United States each year, a little over 5 percent of cases are due to malignant melanoma. Melanoma, unlike the non-melanoma skin cancers, spreads much more easily and accounts for 75 percent of all skin cancer deaths.

Risks and screening

How do you know if you are in the half of the population that is at risk? Everyone is at risk for skin cancer to some degree. Skin cancers occur in Caucasians and African Americans alike though they are less common in African Americans. They can also occur on areas of the body that have never been exposed to the sun. Melanoma is distinguished somewhat from the non-melanoma cancers in that it is linked more strongly to sunburns, especially those experienced early in life, rather than with long-term cumulative exposure to the sun. It is also more common in those with a large number of moles. Risk factors related to all forms of skin cancer include

- having a fair complexion: those with blonde or red hair, blue eyes, and who burn easily are at a higher risk
- having a family or personal history of skin cancer
- having a large number of moles
- living in more tropical regions
- having a history of a severe sunburn in childhood
- spending time at high elevations: risk of skin damage increases at higher altitudes
- working in occupations requiring a lot of time out of doors
- being in environments in which snow and water reflect the sun's rays, increasing the chance of sunburn
- taking some medications, including a few antibiotics, birth control pills, some high blood pressure, anti-inflammatory, diabetic, and depression medications that increase sensitivity to sunlight: risk increases when combined with sun exposure

The odds of survival with melanoma are directly related to the depth of the tumor, making early detection paramount. Melanomas can arise in normal tissue or develop in an existing mole. A mnemonic commonly used to describe the characteristics of melanoma are the ABCDs. This stands for:

A – asymmetry – the two halves of the mole may appear different,

B – border – the edges of the mole can be irregular and notched,

C – color – the color appears uneven unlike a regular mole. This can include shades of black, brown, blue or even pink, red, or white,

D – diameter - the diameter of a melanoma is frequently greater than the size of a pencil eraser (>5mm) In men, melanomas are most commonly found on the head, neck, and trunk. In women, they are found most often on the lower legs.

PREVENTION

Before discussing sun avoidance and risk that our readers will venture outside only when the moon is shining, we need to point out a few benefits of the sun. Life would not exist on earth if it were not for the sun. Sensible sun exposure actually plays a very significant role in cancer *prevention*. A few minutes spent in the sun can provide your body with more vitamin D than can several glasses of milk or a vitamin supplement. Vitamin D, in turn, plays a preventative role not only in osteoporosis, but also in prostate, breast, and colon cancer, cancers with a much higher mortality than all skin cancers combined. An inverse relationship has been noted between sun exposure and thirteen types of cancer. A study published in 2002 estimated that lack of sufficient UVB radiation may account for almost 24,000 cancer deaths each year in the United States, making daily sun exposure an important part of the cancer-prevention lifestyle (Grant, 2002). Those who have had the misfortune of developing melanoma, which kills nearly 8,000 in the U.S. every year, may find this concerning, but moderate, sensible sun exposure actually increases survival from melanoma (Berwick, 2005)!

A few other benefits of spending time outside deserve mention. Outdoor air has fewer toxins than does indoor air, and exercise options expand considerably once you are outside the front door. Time spent in the sun has mental health benefits as well, as those in the north who suffer from seasonal affective disorder through the winter months understand too well. Stress reduction and increased exercise, at least in mice, showed a protective effect against the development of skin cancer.

So, how do we reap the benefits of the sun safely? Our first line of defense should encompass common-sense measures to avoid overexposure. These include avoiding sun exposure during the worst times, between 11am and 3pm. Wearing protective clothing, hats, and using umbrellas can provide significant protection and seems lost to an age when skin cancer was uncommon. Loose fitting, tightly woven fabrics provide the best protection. Clothing such as T-shirts allow the sun to penetrate to a degree and the protection offered is less than that offered by a sunscreen with SPF 15. Do not forget sunglasses. Melanomas can occur on the retina of the eye, and lack of protection raises the risk of cataracts. It is also difficult to apply sunscreen to the tissue surrounding the eyes. Most sunglasses available offer protection against UVA and UVB rays, and the inexpensive variety are usually as good as the pricier varieties. Look for this mention of protection on the label when purchasing sunglasses. Make sure to protect your lips as well. If you are planning a trip south or a day at the beach, you may want to check out the UV index (see Table 4-1). The UV index ranks UV radiation levels on a scale of 1-11+. The Environmental Protection Agency has a Web site where you can find out the UV index at your location based on zip code or city. This can be accessed at www.epa.gov/sunwise/uvindex.html.

The use of a sunscreen with an SPF of 15 or higher is recommended strongly, but the recommendation has generated some questioning recently. The incidence of melanoma has continued to rise in countries where people have adopted widespread use of sunscreens. One explanation is that overdependence on sunscreens may actually increase the risk of melanoma, since people feel protected and spend more time in the sun. Studies have been conflicting, showing both an increase and a decrease in nevi (moles that can turn into melanoma) with the use of sunscreen, depending on the study. Of further concern is that using sunscreen blocks the formation of vitamin D, and some sunscreens contain possible carcinogens that could be absorbed through your skin.

Using sunscreen clearly decreases the risk of sunburns that put a person at risk for skin cancer, and allows one to spend more time in the sun. It has also been shown to decrease the number of *non*-melanoma skin cancers in rodents. Sunscreen preparations have changed over time as well. Originally, sunscreens available in the U.S. only provided protection against UVB rays, but a sunscreen was recently approved by the FDA that offers protection against UVA rays as well. This filter, Mexoryl™SX is owned by L'Oreal and has been used in Europe, Asia and Canada. We hope subsequent studies using this preparation will offer more promising results in the war against skin cancer. Since we do not have solid evidence that sunscreen prevents cancer at this time, it is prudent to keep in mind the common-sense methods of protection in addition to applying the sunscreen. The bottom line is: do not rely on sunscreen alone and exercise common sense.

Table 4-1. UV index

Exposure CATEGORY	UV INDEX	Sun Protection Recommendations
LOW	<2	This is generally safe Wear sunscreen, SPF 15 if you burn easily Wear sunglasses At all exposure levels keep in mind that snow and sand increase your exposure
MODERATE	3-5	Wear sunscreen, SPF 15 Avoid midday sun exposure Wear sunglasses
HIGH	6-7	Wear sunscreen, SPF 15 Avoid midday sun exposure Wear sunglasses Wear a hat; use an umbrella if you will be out at midday
VERY HIGH	8-10	Wear sunscreen, SPF 15 Avoid midday sun exposure Wear sunglasses Wear protective clothing and a hat if you will be out at midday, use an umbrella
EXTREME	11+	Wear sunscreen, SPF 15 Avoid midday sun exposure Wear sunglasses Wear protective clothing and a hat and seek shade if you will be out at midday, use an umbrella if shade is not available

Tanning beds

Teenagers now model a bronze glamour from tanning salons that their parents achieved a generation ago with baby oil and aluminum foil. Is there evidence that an "electric" tan is safer? First, there is no such thing as a safe tan. Long-term exposure to natural OR artificial sources of ultraviolet rays increases the risk of developing skin cancer. The sun's rays consist of ultraviolet A (UVA) and ultraviolet B (UVB) rays. Manufacturers of tanning beds claim the "safety" of the salon tan is due to the form of ultraviolet rays present. Tanning beds are roughly 95 percent UVA and 5 percent UVB, with UVB rays having been considered the "dangerous rays." The truth is, both UVA and UVB rays cause skin damage. UVA rays take longer to damage the skin, but penetrate deeper. The implication of this is uncertain at this time. It does raise our eyebrows slightly that the melanocytes (the cells that manufacture melanin, the pigment that causes our skin to become "tan") are in these deeper layers. Melanocytes are the cells that, when damaged, can develop into melanoma. In one study, women who used tanning beds more than once a month were 55 percent more likely to develop malignant melanoma than were those that didn't (Veierod, 2003). In addition, the use of tanning beds to "pre-tan" before traveling south is not recommended and could be detrimental. A tan produced by artificial sunlight does not provide as much protection against UV sun damage as does one provided by natural sunlight, and can give a false impression of safety.

The FDA has approved sunless tanning products in the form of lotions, which color the skin with a dye. Although they appear to be safe, we still caution that these products have not been available long enough to know their safety for certain, and there is potential for the chemicals to be absorbed through the skin as well. In addition, these are approved for external use only and concern has been raised that the whole body sprays done in salons could result in absorption through the eyes, nose, and mouth. These areas should be protected if a whole-body spray is desired. Tanning pills can also be found. These are not safe, period.

Electromagnetic Fields

The jury is still out concerning the effects of electromagnetic fields (EMFs) on health and cancer risk. All of us are exposed to EMFs emitted from a range of objects from power lines to cell phones, and this exposure is one of the most rapidly expanding environmental influences in our lives. Electric fields are easily shielded, whereas magnetic fields pass through most materials and are more difficult to shield. Both decrease rapidly as the distance from the source increases. Several studies have shown cancer risk increases with magnetic field exposure, but this is not the case with electric fields. Magnetic fields are described by their frequency. Examples of extremely low frequency magnetic fields include those from power lines and household appliances. High frequency electromagnetic fields are generated by cell phones and radio and television broadcasts.

High voltage power lines

Concern over exposure to high voltage power lines was raised when, in 1972, a study in Colorado demonstrated that children who died from leukemia were two to three times more likely to have lived within 131 feet of a high current electrical transmission or distribution line. Another study done in England and Wales showed a significant increase in childhood leukemia in children that were born within 600 meters, and more so within 200 meters of high voltage, overhead power lines (Draper, 2005). Many studies have been conducted worldwide since that time with mixed results, some showing no evidence for concern. If you are looking for a home and all else is equal, choose the one that puts a greater distance between your children and high voltage power lines.

Household appliances

As with high voltage power lines, the linkage between cancer and EMFs from household appliances has not been conclusively proven or refuted. A study in *Epidemiology* did show an association between common household appliances and cancer risk. Children whose mothers used electric blankets or mattress pads while pregnant and children that used them had an increased risk of acute lymphoblastic leukemia. There was also an increased cancer risk in children who used hair dryers, video machines in arcades, and video games connected to a TV. While distance from the TV did not seem to carry much risk, the amount of time children spent watching television was linked to their risk of developing leukemia (Hatch, 1998). With obesity in children increasing and test scores declining, this offers yet another reason to limit your child's TV-watching time! In general, exposure to electromagnetic fields in daily life probably does not contribute significantly to adult cancer risk. A few general precautions are suggested, especially in the case of pregnant women and children:

- Keep children away from the sides and back of computer monitors where emissions are the highest.
- When buying a new computer monitor, purchase the low emission type.
- Keep clock radios at least three feet from your bed.
- Sit back at least five feet from the TV, avoiding the sides and back.
- Stay three feet away from the microwave oven when in use.
- Turn off electric blankets and mattresses prior to retiring and limit their use to only the coldest of nights.

Again, it is worthy to note that electromagnetic fields drop off very rapidly with distance from the source. Further research is needed to see if there are truly any concerns related to EMFs and if a cause and effect relationship exists. If you or your child occasionally stands next to the microwave or is seated a foot from the TV, do not be an alarmist. The stress from being overly zealous about little exposures is probably more dangerous than the exposure!

Cell phones

While a rumor some time ago claimed that the use of cell phones may increase the risk of developing brain tumors, the majority of studies to date do not support this. A retrospective study done in Sweden did show an increase in acoustic neuromas (benign brain tumors involving the auditory nerve) in analog cell phone users with use over a ten-year period, but this was not seen with non-analogue cell phones (Lonn, 2004). Prolonged exposure to cell phones was also found to raise brain temperature in animals, but the clinical significance of this is unknown. "Cordless" phones that have a base unit operate at much lower power levels and have not been part of this concern.

As discussed in the preceding chapter, many causes of cancer, such as smoking, have a latency period of fifteen to twenty years or more before any correlation with cancer is found. We need not be alarmists with the reassuring studies to date, but may want to consider how concerns about cell phone use have been addressed in Europe. As a precaution, government agencies in Britain, France, and Germany have recommended that children use cell phones only for essential calls since their brains are still developing.

The FDA suggests that people who are concerned but want to use cell phones use the phones for shorter conversations or when a conventional phone is not available. They also recommend a headset to place more distance between the antenna and the phone user. Placing phones on a belt has not been evaluated, but does raise some additional concern, given the proximity to the ovaries and prostate. Practice common sense, especially while on the road, and if a "land" phone is available, use it first. Consider purchasing a headset. Limit use by children and teens as a precaution. If cell phones turn out to be completely safe in thirty years, you may have at least prevented an auto accident!

It is important to discard old cell phones carefully when you are through with them. Some cell phones contain cadmium, beryllium, arsenic, and antimony, which are known carcinogens. If you have questions about how to recycle your old phones, you can check the Web site www.donateaphone.com. This site also offers information on general cell phone safety and etiquette.

Home Exposures

"All of us face a variety of risks to our health as we go about our day-to-day lives...Indoor air pollution is one risk that you can do something about."

—U.S. Environmental Protection Agency

We view our homes as havens, as places to retreat to from the chaos of the world, places we are safe. We think of pollution as something outdoors, occurring in the big cities. Broadcasting segments about the fact that indoor air pollution in the cleanest, best-maintained homes is worse than the air outside would not improve ratings for the news stations we tune into after a long day out in the world. Exposure to harmful substances, some that contribute to cancer risk, in our homes, is disconcerting at best.

At the risk of darkening scenes of a blissful mother holding her child by the fireplace or playing on the swing set, we hope to present a few cautions—nothing revolutionary—that could possibly make long-term differences in the health of you and your family. We preface this by a simple prevention idea to remind the reader we are not "sitting ducks" awaiting massacre by carcinogens; we have a lot we can do to minimize the risks at hand. As you read this, adopt a mindset of optimism, and have fun with how easy avoiding some exposures can be. At the end of this chapter, we present a list of common household products of concern, followed by a list of alternative products that may be safer.

Houseplants

As "glass-half-full" individuals, we wish to start this list with a simple remedy for confronting a few of the toxins in our home environment. Thanks to research done by NASA, we do have a solution for eliminating some of the toxins in our homes. Dr. B. Wolvertson, a NASA scientist, has performed extensive research on the role of houseplants in improving indoor air quality. His research has evaluated the ability of several common houseplants to remove common household carcinogens from the air (Wolverton, 1997).

Three of the most common indoor air pollutants that can cause cancer include

- formaldehyde – found in pressed wood, particle board, air fresheners, permanent press clothing, wallpaper, upholstery
- benzene – found in wood stain and varnishes, paint stripper, motor oil, driveway sealer, automotive cleaners, weed killer
- trichloroethylene - found in adhesives, paints, varnishes, paint strippers, pesticides

In studies, formaldehyde was best removed by the heartleaf philodendron, spider plant, and golden pothos; benzene, by gerbera daisy and chrysanthemum (see Table 4-2). Other good houseplant choices include Chinese evergreen, English ivy, peace lily, marginata, and warnecki. If you are wondering about the number of plants to have in your home, the magic number for decreasing airborne carcinogens appeared to be roughly fifteen plants in six inch or greater containers per 2000 square feet of floor space.

A quick word of caution about purchasing plants to improve your indoor air. Over-watering plants can result in mold production, which can cause allergies in some people. In addition, many houseplants are toxic to curious pets and crawling children, so choose non-poisonous varieties if you have little ones or herbivorous pets.

Table 4-2. Houseplants To Remove Carcinogens

Formaldehyde	Boston fern, spider plant, palms, rubber plant, English ivy, Janet Craig, chrysanthemum, philodendron, peace lily, golden pathos
Benzene	Spider plant, peace lily, gerbera daisy, chrysanthemum
Trichlorethylene	Ficus, parlor palm

Home and Garden Pesticides

According to several studies, the use of home and garden pesticides is associated with up to a seven-fold increased risk of leukemia and lymphoma in children under the age of ten (Menegaux, 2006; Buckley, 2000; Ma, 2002, others). By pesticides, we mean to include indoor and outdoor gardening chemicals, insecticides including bug spray and shampoos to treat head lice, fertilizers, herbicides, and fungicides. A child who is exposed to professional pest services (even though they have guidelines where, based on the age of children, they recommend children leaving the home for various periods) is three times more likely to develop non-Hodgkin's lymphoma than a non-exposed child (Buckley, 2000). As would be expected, the duration and frequency of exposures increases risk. Risk is also greatest to children who are exposed in utero. If you must use pesticides or insecticides, practice a few protective measures:

- Use goggles, a mask (fume mask), and gloves.
- Wear protective clothing. Remove them before entering your home and wash immediately, separate from other clothing. Always remove your shoes before entering your home to avoid tracking in chemicals.
- Do not use pesticides on windy days.
- Keep children away when applying pesticides, insecticides, or other chemicals.

In addition, if you need the services of an exterminator, choose a professional pest service that practices integrated pest management (IPM).

Several commercial lawn companies post signs that warn people to keep dogs off the grass after it is fertilized: studies show an increased risk of cancer in exposed dogs. Practice the same precautions with children! If you do fertilize, wait until after a good soaking rain before allowing your children to walk on the grass. If you struggle with weeds in your lawn, look for alternatives to common weed killers containing 2,4-Dichlorophenoxyacetic acid. Dogs exposed to this are twice as likely to die from cancer than those who are not (Hayes, 1991). Why do we present information on dogs? It is felt that dogs are at greater risk than are humans, because they have more contact with the grass. A child crawling or somersaulting through the yard would have significant contact as well. Alternatives to weed killer include hand-pulling weeds, using very hot water to kill them, or learning to tolerate a few weeds in your yard. If the weeds continue to bother you, consider rock gardens or other forms of landscaping.

"Weeds are flowers too, once you get to know them."

—Eeyore, from A.A. Milne's "Winnie the Pooh"

Water

If you have city water you probably do not need to have it tested, although we still recommend using a filter. If you have well water, have it tested. Carcinogens have been found in well water near the authors' homes where one would least expect it. The use of well water has been linked in various studies to an increased risk of lung, bladder, kidney, and colorectal cancer. Common contaminants in well water include atrazine, arsenic, lead, radium, and volatile organic compounds (VOCs).

Filters can lower your risk of exposure and can eliminate chlorine. Most common filters do not filter out microorganisms, and those people with weakened immune systems should avoid well water altogether. Well water can also be the source of infection from the bacteria *H. pylori,* an organism that is strongly linked with stomach cancer and is discussed further in Chapter Six. *H. pylori* is present in around 65 percent of private well water samples. This is not a concern with public water supplies, since chlorine eliminates the bacteria.

The chlorination process illustrates an important concept in cancer prevention. Carcinogens are produced in the chlorination process and have been the cause of concern in some health circles. The virtues of chlorination, however, far outweigh its negative aspects. With the elimination of *H. pylori* from our drinking water through chlorination, we have likely prevented many cases of stomach cancer.

When choosing a filter we recommend purchasing a reverse-osmosis system to use in your kitchen for drinking water and cooking. If you are building a new home, investing in a pump will allow you to have purified water in multiple areas of your home and make the water stream stronger, but is fairly pricey to install in an existing home. Adding a chlorine filter to your showerhead can also reduce your exposure to chlorine that can be absorbed through the skin, and chloroform gas, which occurs when hot water from the shower containing chlorine is exposed to air.

PETS

Animals can be wonderful companions for adults and children alike. Teaching children to care for animals can instruct them in important life lessons. As animal lovers ourselves, we hope to shed light on a few concerns that can be easily addressed with a little knowledge.

Flea collars and flea products often contain ingredients that have been linked with the development of childhood brain cancer (Pogoda, 1997). Most indoor pets do not suffer from flea problems unless present before they were adopted, but outdoor pets frequently pick up these tiny pests. If your pet does contract fleas, conservative measures can help combat the attack. Frequent vacuuming to remove flea eggs, combing pets with flea combs, and washing pet bedding frequently are vitally important. Bathing is important as well, and most shampoos kill fleas.

Other non-toxic measures for dealing with fleas include flea traps and biological controls such as nematodes watered into your lawn. Some herbal treatments are available as well, but the authors are uncertain of the success rate of these. If you must use conventional flea treatments, practice extra caution. Never let children handle a pet wearing a flea collar. If you do use flea bombs, wear a fume mask, goggles, and gloves, and make sure no one, especially children, are allowed in the home for an extended period afterwards.

Although it is unlikely, the subject of whether feline leukemia virus in cats can be transmitted to children, especially in utero, has been the subject of some controversy in the past. Happily, there is a vaccine for cats that can prevent feline leukemia and eliminate any potential risk. For those who are concerned about keeping kitty while pregnant, this is a simple solution. If cost is a concern, it is even possible now to order vaccinations for pets online and to self-administer the injection. Taking the time and effort to immunize your feline also gives greater hope that kitty will grow old with baby rather than succumb to the virus!

There is not a vaccine available for toxoplasmosis, an infection (which causes birth defects not cancer) that can be acquired while changing cat litter, and pregnant women still need to exercise caution. Cat litter can also be a concern. Crystalline silica is a known carcinogen and is found in several cat litters. One of the authors used to recommend women have someone else change the litter box during pregnancy!

In addition, many puppies are plagued with worms, some of which can be transmitted to humans. The safety of anti-worm medications for pregnant women has not been established and a non-pregnant partner should gather samples if there is a concern.

Wood burning stoves and fireplaces

According to the Environmental Protection Agency (EPA), wood smoke contains volatile organic compounds (VOCs), some of which are cancer causing. This has become an increasing environmental concern, and a few cities in northern California have even adopted some form of ban on wood burning stoves and fireplaces in new construction. They do continue to allow low-polluting wood stoves and inserts in fireplaces approved by the EPA, as well as fireplaces fueled by natural gas. If you are building, consider opting for a natural gas fireplace. If you have an existing wood burning fireplace, see if updating this to a natural gas version is within your budget. If you do use a wood burning fireplace or stove, the EPA offers the following recommendations to avoid the release of toxic chemicals:

- Never burn coated, painted, or pressure-treated wood.
- Never burn garbage or cardboard, since plastics and colored inks in these can release harmful chemicals.
- Never burn plywood, driftwood, particleboard, or any wood with glue in it.

For further information about wood stoves and fireplace safety, you can check out www.epa.gov/woodstoves/efficiently.html.

Kerosene heaters should be avoided as well, since these release formaldehyde vapors into the air.

Location, location, location

Real estate agents claim that location is the number one factor in choosing a home, and from a cancer perspective, location makes a difference as well. Some locations have been said to predispose residents to developing cancer. Female residents in counties near nuclear reactors were feared to have an elevated risk of developing breast cancer at one time, however a survey conducted by the National Cancer Institute demonstrated that if there was such a risk, it was too small to be detected by the study methods (Jablon, 1991). Other areas that may carry risk, such as those near heavy traffic areas, have not been as widely publicized.

Automobile emissions are known to be carcinogenic due to exhaust gases as well as brake-block rubbing off. Many studies have shown an increase in cancer rates in people living in high-density traffic areas, especially in children. A recent study in Great Britain revealed evidence that 24 percent of childhood cancers in the study area were attributable to early life proximity to railway stations, bus stations, ferry terminals, railways, and roads. Of these, roads posed the greatest risk (Knox, 2006). For those mentally calculating the mileage from their home to the nearest region of high-density traffic, three kilometers was the distance from busy roads at which there no longer appeared to be a risk. While specific distances were not studied in the case of oil refineries, exposure to petrochemicals in regions near these refineries has been linked with an increase in developing leukemia in young adults (Yu, 2006).

Cancer clusters (several cases of cancer beyond that expected by chance occurring in a region) have occurred in many regions. Some of these have been traced to a particular exposure, such as contaminated well water; many others do not have an identifiable cause, or may have occurred by coincidence. Although there are many issues to consider when choosing a home, if you are moving to an unfamiliar area, and time and energy permit, you may want to look into whether or not any questions about cancer clusters have been raised. In addition, you may want to check out the TRI database discussed earlier in the general precautions section. The Web site URL is listed in the resources at the end of this chapter.

Dry-cleaning

Avoid dry-cleaning clothes if possible, and if they cannot be cleaned at home, explore other alternatives. Studies have shown that workers in drycleaners have a higher incidence of several types of cancer, particularly esophageal cancer, than do people at large. The primary solvent used in dry-cleaning is perchloroethylene (perc), which has been found to cause cancer in rats and mice. In 1995, the International Agency for Research on Cancer (IARC) labeled perc as probably carcinogenic to humans as well.

A safer alternative is available if your clothes cannot be laundered at home. "Wet cleaning" uses water rather than chemical solvents. To see if this is available in your area, check the Environmental Protection Agencies Web site at www.epa.gov/dfe/pubs/garment/gcrg/cleanguide.pdf, which lists places where wet cleaning is available. Wet cleaning has been used for many years in England with satisfactory results.

If you do take clothes to the drycleaners, hang them in a closet or area distant from your bedroom for several days before wearing them. If they smell of chemicals, bring them back and ask to have them recleaned.

Air fresheners

Do air fresheners actually make our homes fresher? Some air fresheners contain baking soda, which can neutralize and absorb odors. Most air fresheners, however, either interfere with your ability to smell odors by coating your nasal passages with an oil film, or by releasing a nerve-deadening agent that acts on your nasal passages so you can no longer smell the odor you wish to avoid.

Researchers at the Environmental Protection Agency state that potentially harmful smog could build up inside of homes through the reactions caused by plug-in (electric) air fresheners and ozone. This reaction creates formaldehyde, a carcinogen. Ozone is present in homes and is produced by vehicle exhaust reacting with sunlight: it is thus more concerning in urban areas and heavy traffic areas.

Knowing this, are non-electric air fresheners safer alternatives? Many air fresheners contain known carcinogens including formaldehyde and paradichlorobenzene, a pesticide and potential carcinogen. Several of these come in aerosol containers and the size of aerosol-propelled particles allows easier absorption into the lungs and bloodstream.

Alternatives to air fresheners that are non-toxic are available. For carpet odors, try spreading baking soda on the odor and vacuuming after several minutes (first test this on an inconspicuous area to avoid stains). Good ventilation, opening the windows, using exhaust fans, banning smoking in your home, and simmering lemons and water on the stove can provide relief from annoying smells as well.

Outdoor play sets and other pressure-treated wood

Wooden play sets, picnic tables, decks, and gardens by the fence bring healthy, happy thoughts to most Americans, especially those who have to wait for the summer months to venture outside. The greenish tinge to wood products indicates they will not rot within a few seasons; however, this should not conjure up the healthy image green otherwise depicts. This green hue is a visual clue that the wood was pressure treated with arsenic, a known carcinogen, to increase its lifespan. Until it was banned for use in decks and play sets by the Environmental Protection Agency in 2003, CCA (chromated copper arsenate) was used in roughly 90 percent of lumber designed for outdoor purposes. The Environmental Working Group has estimated that 1 in 500 children, a haunting statistic, will develop cancer later in life directly from their time spent on pressure-treated wood structures.

While CCA-treated wood has been banned, many structures in playgrounds and back yards built prior to 2003 will last many years because of CCA. Unlike those of many chemicals, arsenic levels do not decrease substantially over time and older structures still pose a risk. In addition, retail stores may still carry CCA-treated wood purchased prior to 2003. To reduce risks of exposure, children should wash their hands after playing on wooden play sets, and any surface on which food is served, such as picnic tables, should be covered with a tablecloth. It is also advisable to seal these structures with polyurethane every six months, or at least yearly in the northern states. Staying away from soil under CCA-treated wood decks and avoiding gardening near CCA-treated fences is encouraged as well.

If you elect to dispose of CCA-treated wood, do not burn it. It is illegal to burn CCA-treated wood in all fifty states. Burning does not remove arsenic and a single twelve foot long 2-by-6 contains enough arsenic to kill 200 adults!

The Environmental Working Group has an informative site with ten tips for parents concerned about exposure in their children. This is accessible at www.ewg.org/issues/arsenic/10tips.php. There are also test kits available to test the arsenic content that can rub off on tiny hands or leak into soil below decks and play sets. These are available at www.ewg.org/reports/poisonwoodrivals/orderform.php.

Bug spray

A recent study showed that children exposed to bug spray during their mothers' pregnancies and in early childhood had double the risk of developing acute leukemia (Menegaux, 2006). If we skip the spray, how do we survive the onslaught of mosquitos that are the hallmark of American summers for many of us? The mosquito is so ubiquitous that many residents of Minnesota, where one of the authors resides, wear T-shirts with a mosquito depicted as the state bird!

Alternatives are available, but first we must caution that these recommendations are only for those people in areas free from malaria and without concern over arboviruses. If you live in an area where malaria is endemic, the risk that bug spray poses doesn't stand up to the benefits. Worldwide, a child dies every thirty seconds from malaria, a disease that is transmitted by mosquitos. There are few chemicals, especially those that would be approved for use in an insect spray, that could cause such devastation. Within the United States, exposure to equine encephalitis and West Nile virus can pose concerns, and the liberal use of bug spray would similarly be warranted.

DEET is currently by far the most effective repellent available, capable of repelling mosquitos for about five hours. Overall, toxicity studies with DEET have shown it to have a good safety profile, considering the number of people that have used this and the time it has been available (forty years).

Alternatives that have been investigated are an option where bites are primarily a nuisance, although most have a short duration of action. Citronella-based bug spray (such as Natropel®, etc.) work well short-term (twenty minutes or less) and can be reapplied. Soybean oil (Bite Blocker®, etc.) protects for around ninety minutes. Eucalyptus-oil-based repellents (such as Repel Lemon Eucalyptus®, etc.) are probably the most promising plant-based repellents and can protect for up to four hours. The popular alternative (Skin So Soft® by Avon), which has been recommended for pregnant women and small children, does offer protection, but only for about ten minutes. Other plant-based repellents and DEET-impregnated wrist bands do not appear to offer any significant protection. In addition, several of these probably do not offer protection against other insects, such as ticks, as DEET does.

Common-sense methods should be exercised first, no matter your location. Avoid being outside at dusk. Wear clothing that protects you from bites. At a barbeque, burn a citronella candle. When you do apply bug spray, try applying the majority to your clothes, hat, and hair to minimize contact with your skin. This, however, requires protective clothing, since the repellent in most bug sprays works primarily where it is sprayed and the effectiveness drops off rapidly with distance. Find ways to reduce the mosquito population near your home as well. Avoid sources of standing water such as empty barrels and buckets that can be mosquito breeding grounds. If your neighborhood is being sprayed for mosquitos, leave for the day.

Asbestos

Exposure to asbestos is primarily an occupational exposure, but we list it here for those who may have asbestos in their homes and consider "do-it-yourself" projects. Breathing in asbestos is strongly linked with lung cancer and an otherwise rare form of lung cancer called mesothelioma, a tumor involving the lining of the lungs. The risk of developing these cancers is exponentially increased if those exposed also smoke. If you are considering any remodeling, check the date your home was built. Asbestos was banned from use in homes in 1970.

If your home was built prior to 1970 and has asbestos insulation, do not be overly alarmed. There is virtually no risk from asbestos products **if** they are left intact and not changed, damaged, or disturbed. If you decide to remodel or have asbestos removed, hire a qualified contractor. In this case, we also recommend you contact the Environmental Protection Agencies Toxic Substances Control Act

(TSCA) assistance line at 1-202-554-1414, or visit the office of Pollution Prevention and Toxic Substances' asbestos home page at www.epa.gov/asbestos.

When organizing your home you may also want to consider discarding products that could contain asbestos. Examples of these include asbestos gloves, old stovetop covers, and older ironing board covers.

Carpet cleaning

If you have your carpets cleaned or clean them yourselves, read the labels on cleaning solutions. The chemicals perchloroethylene and 1-1-1 trichlorothane found in some spot removers and carpet cleaners have been shown to cause cancer in animals. Also, be aware that some carpet protectors have been removed from the market. Despite this, one of the authors was recently offered one of these products since the company still had a "good supply" left over. To decrease your need for carpet cleaning, adopt a "no-shoes-in-the-home" policy to help keep your carpets clean. This will also decrease the number of "unseen" chemicals brought into your home on your shoes from the outside. When choosing new carpeting, look for the green CRI carpet testing program label that signifies the carpet and glues meet industry standards. Ask the installer to air out the carpet for a few days prior to installation, and open doors and windows, and use exhaust fans when it is installed.

Mothballs

Mothballs frequently contain the known carcinogens naphthalene and paradichlororbenzene. Exposure to mothballs has been linked to an increased risk of developing non-Hodgkin's lymphoma. If you struggle with moths, an excellent alternative is using cedar planks.

Pressed wood products

Many pressed wood products contain formaldehyde, a known carcinogen. Fiberboard, frequently used for furniture tops, cabinets, and drawer fronts, tends to be the highest in formaldehyde content. Other wood products that may contain formaldehyde include particleboard and hardwood plywood paneling. It may be worth investing in more expensive but cleaner, solid wood products. If you do purchase these products, review the houseplants listed at the beginning of this chapter that can absorb formaldehyde in addition to decorating your new furnishings. Sealing these products with water-based polyurethane can also decrease emissions.

Exposures in the garage

Practicing good ventilation is particularly important while working in the garage. Petroleum hydrocarbons found in gasoline and motor oils are associated with lung and skin cancer. Some petroleum distillates also contain benzene, a strong carcinogen.

Do-it-yourself projects

Do-it-yourself projects can save money and provide personal satisfaction, but make sure you invest the time and money to do this safely. Always read product labels, use gloves with chemicals, a mask where indicated, and dispose of hazardous materials safely. It may cost more to hire someone, but part of that cost may be for the training it takes to do those projects safely.

Caution should be used if you will be working with wood and exposed to **wood dust,** which has been labeled a human carcinogen. There is a strong association between occupational exposure to wood dust and cancers of the sinuses and nasal cavities. More recently, associations have been made between wood dust exposure and lung cancer. Many do-it-your-selfers are exposed to wood dust outside of the workplace when sanding and cutting wood. For these projects, we recommend using a HEPA mask. Remember to use this during clean-up as well, since this may present the greatest exposure. A HEPA mask is also recommended when sanding walls that have been painted, since aluminum silicate, which may be carcinogenic when dry, is present in some paint.

Products such as **spray paint, paint removers**, and some **wood stains** may contain methylene chloride, a chemical known to cause breast cancer in animals. If you need to use products with methylene chloride, invest in a mask approved for exposure to vapors. Always use these products in well-ventilated spaces and never indoors if possible. Use a fume mask approved for vapors, as well as gloves and protective clothing if you **seal coat** your driveway yourself. Blacktop driveway sealer contains chemicals known to cause cancer according to California's Proposition 65 (see Appendix C). If you have this done professionally, keep windows closed and try to leave for the day. Do not allow your children to play on the driveway for several days after the sealing and wear proper footwear. If you can afford concrete instead of asphalt when laying a driveway, consider this for the health as well as maintenance advantages.

Adhesives

If you enjoy activities, such as building models, that require the use of adhesives, read labels and practice the same caution that would be enforced in an industrial setting. Many adhesives contain chemicals that have been shown to be carcinogenic.

Personal Product Exposures

"An average adult is exposed to over 100 unique chemicals in personal-care products every day. These exposures add up."

—Jane Houlihan

Talcum powder

Application of talc below the waist has been associated with a particular form of ovarian cancer. Find an alternative.

Hair color

The conclusion on whether or not hair dyes raise the risk of developing cancer is unsettled. Studies have shown a significantly increased risk of non-Hodgkins lymphoma in women exposed to dark color hair dyes. This increase was seen only in women who began using hair dyes before 1980; used permanent rather than non-permanent dyes; chose dark colors such as brown, black, and red; and used them at least eight times per year for twenty-five years. Studies that are more recent show only a small link between hair dye and the risk of leukemia and multiple myeloma (Zhang, 2005). One study showed an increase in bladder cancer in people genetically predisposed, but this is not practical to screen for in the average individual (Gago-Dominguez, 2003). Carcinogens are present in the majority of currently available hair dyes, but the chemical content may not be the issue and this needs further evaluation. Hair dyes cause a chemical reaction to change the color of hair, and concern could lie in the reaction or products produced.

Using hair color is a personal choice and issues other than cancer prevention are present! If you do choose to use hair dyes, especially dark hair dyes, consider decreasing the frequency of use. In addition, you may want to investigate the alternatives available, such as using henna.

Deodorants/Antiperspirants

It is controversial, though unlikely, that the use of deodorants and antiperspirants contribute to breast cancer, but if a natural product that does not contain parabens or aluminum is effective, use it. In a study published in a European cancer journal, the frequency and earlier onset of antiperspirant/deodorant usage with underarm shaving was associated with an earlier age of breast cancer (McGrath, 2003). A preservative (parabens) used in deodorants and antiperspirants mimics the activity of estrogen. Since estrogen accelerates the growth of breast cancer cells, some researchers have suggested that the use of these could cause the accumulation of paraben in breast tissue and subsequently lead to cancer. One study did find parabens in tissue from most breast cancers but whether or not this is related to the cancers is questionable (Darbre, 2004). Other studies have not demonstrated any risk from deodorants, antiperspirants, or early underarm shaving and if these do pose a risk, it is probably minimal.

Baby products

Read labels on the baby products you use. Some preservatives, such as quaternium 15 and bronopol, break down to release formaldehyde, a carcinogen. With products such as teethers, bath books, and bath toys look for products marked "phthalate free," since phthalates are frequently not listed on the label. Phthalates are a group of chemicals used in plastics to improve flexibility. In Europe, three types of phthalates have been banned from use in childrens' products, and three others have been banned in products designed for children under the age of three. California is evaluating a similar ban.

Around-Town Exposures

The gas station

It is well documented that exposure to gasoline fumes raises the risk of developing cancer. Many gasoline pumps carry warnings of this danger. Men who work near gasoline products have a significantly increased risk of developing male breast cancer, but studies of women in this setting are lacking (Hansen, 2000). Stay in your car with the windows up while fueling. Fill your tank completely if possible to limit your exposure and trips to the gas station. Do not try to add extra fuel by pumping the nozzle once it stops. According to the Environmental Protection Agency (EPA), "topping off" your gas tank is bad for your health and the environment, and actually costs more! Fill your tank and replace the nozzle immediately when done. If you are pregnant, consider having someone else go to the gas station for you.

Golfing

If you love to golf, check on the pesticides your golf course uses on their greens. Golf course supervisors have elevated risks of non-Hodgkin's lymphoma, brain, prostate, and lung cancers (Kross, 1996). You do not want your passion to put you at risk, nor do you want the people making the course beautiful for you to suffer the consequences. If you enjoy golfing, remove your shoes after playing and before entering your home to avoid tracking in chemicals. Also, wash your hands thoroughly after touching golf balls and never lick or kiss them!

Occupational Exposures

"I know there are troubles of more than one kind.
Some come from ahead and some come from behind.
But I've brought a big bat. I'm all ready you see.
Now my troubles are going to have troubles with me!"

—Dr. Seuss

While a thorough review of occupational exposures is beyond the scope of this book, the principles we discussed earlier in this chapter apply to the workplace as well. We hope that a bat will not be necessary to chase away carcinogens, but the careful use of gloves, masks, proper ventilation, and an understanding of substances you are exposed to at your place of employment can not be overstated.

The first documented cases of cancers due to occupational exposure were noted in 1567, based on observations in Austrian mines. Theophrastus Bombastus von Hohenheim (better known by the name Paracelsus) described the "wasting disease of miners." He is the first to consider a chemical compound as an occupational carcinogen. Currently, roughly 40,000 new cases of cancer per year in the U.S. are attributed to occupational exposures. Apparently, Americans find this acceptable, since the authors have not seen this covered to the degree that hurricanes and terrorism have been, things that have killed far fewer people. Five percent of men and one percent of women will develop cancer in their lifetimes as a result of exposure to carcinogenic substances in their work environment.

If you are exposed to chemicals at work, make sure to review the Material Safety Data Sheets (MSDS) of the chemicals you work with. Employers are required to provide these for each chemical with which their employees work. If you feel uncomfortable, are not informed about the dangers of chemicals at work, or feel you are being subjected to dangerous exposures you can contact OSHA. OSHA has a 24-hour access line available for reporting unsafe work practices at 1-800-321-6742.

In Table 4-3 we discuss a few of the more common occupational risks. We also wish to mention a few occupational exposures because they are related to volunteering or not obviously addressed in employment manuals.

Firefighters

Firefighters, especially in small communities, frequently volunteer their time to protect us in addition to working their regular employment. Firefighters have an increased risk of developing several cancers, including brain, kidney, and bladder cancers as well as non-Hodgkin's lymphoma and leukemia. Those who are not firefighters can help decrease this risk by avoiding PBDE (polybrominated-diphenyl ether)-treated plastics when possible. PBDE is a flame retardant that results in very toxic, carcinogenic compounds when burned. The Swedish based store IKEA has banned this in their products for this reason.

Copy machines

Try to avoid the exhaust when working around copy machines. Copy machines can cause the formation of ozone (possibly a carcinogen), and toner is a possible carcinogen as well. If you are in charge of purchasing paper, choose chlorine-free paper. There is research showing a link between chlorinated products and breast cancer. When chlorinated products are produced or incinerated, dioxin, a carcinogen, is released. Products that are chlorine-free carry the indication that they are PCF, which stands for "processed chlorine free."

Asbestos

If you are exposed to asbestos on the job, absolutely do not smoke. The combination of smoking and asbestos exposure poses a risk for developing cancer much greater than would be expected from that associated with smoking and asbestos exposure alone.

Table 4-3. Cancers Associated with Various Occupational Exposures

Cancers Associated with Various Occupational Exposures		
CANCER	SUBSTANCE OR PROCESS	WORKERS AT RISK
Lung	Natural fibers like wood dust, silica, asbestos. Metals including beryllium, cadmium, chromium compounds, nickel and nickel refining, aluminum production, arsenic dusts and processing arsenic-containing ore, foundry substances, uranium mining, arsenical pesticides, coal gasification, soots, tars, oils, acrylonitrile, petrochemicals and combustion by-products such as polycyclic aromatic hydrocarbons (PAHs), diesel fumes, second-hand smoke, strontium chloride, radon, reactive chemicals including bis (chloromethyl) ether and mustard gas, vinyl chloride, solvents including benzene and toluene.	Painters, printers, chemists. Sandblasting, masonry work, ceramics, glass manufacturing, ship building, metal working including iron and steel foundry work, bar tending, uranium mining, railroad work, truck driving, workers preparing anion exchange resins. Asbestos workers who don't smoke are seven times more likely to die of lung cancer. Asbestos workers who smoke are 50-90 times more likely to develop lung cancer.

Cancers Associated with Various Occupational Exposures		
CANCER	**SUBSTANCE OR PROCESS**	**WORKERS AT RISK**
Bladder	Tetrachloroethylene (PCE), aromatic amines including beta naphthalamine and benzidine, aluminum production, petrochemicals and combustion by-products including polycyclic aromatic hydrocarbons (PAHs) and diesel exhaust, PAHs in coal tars and pitches, arsenic, auramine and magenta dye, rubber processing, leather processing, 4-aminobiphenyl, permanent hair dye, printing.	Dry-cleaning workers, workers involved in the manufacture and use of dyes, including hair colorists (prior to changes in dyes used), leather processing, truck drivers, workers in the rubber industry, metal workers, printing.
Nasal cavities and sinuses	Formaldehyde, isopropyl alcohol manufacture, radium, nickel refining, leather processing, wood processing, chlorophenols, mustard gas, chromates, nickel, strontium chloride.	Radium processors, dial printing, nickel refining, leather processing, wood processing (woodworking, cabinet making, furniture making, sawmill workers, carpentry), shoe manufacturing.

Cancers Associated with Various Occupational Exposures		
CANCER	**SUBSTANCE OR PROCESS**	**WORKERS AT RISK**
Laryngeal	Asbestos, wood dust, paint fumes, metal working fluids and mineral oils, sulfuric acids, mustard gas, isopropyl alcohol, mustard gas, nickel refining.	Metal and construction workers, isopropyl alcohol manufacturing via the strong acid process, mustard gas manufacturing, rubber industry workers, wood working, painting. Tobacco and heavy alcohol intake increase the risk of these cancers by up to 100 times.
Pharynx	Formaldehyde, mustard gas.	Mustard gas manufacturing, embalming.
Mesothelioma (type of lung cancer)	Asbestos.	Construction, fire fighting.
Lymphomas, leukemia, multiple myeloma	Organic solvents including benzene, trichloroethylene (TCE), tetrachloroethylene (PCE), carbon tetrachloride, pesticides, styrene, dioxin, PCBs, hair dyes (especially dark colors prior to 1980), reactive chemicals like butadiene and ethylene oxide.	Laundry and dry-cleaning workers, woodworking, chemists, hair colorists, petroleum and rubber industry workers, leather working, farming, firefighting, aircraft maintenance, roofing, healthcare workers involved with radiation and chemotherapy.

Cancers Associated with Various Occupational Exposures		
CANCER	**SUBSTANCE OR PROCESS**	**WORKERS AT RISK**
Skin	Arsenic, mineral oils, sun exposure, coal tars, polycyclic aromatic hydrocarbons (PAHs), ionizing radiation.	Outdoor occupations (construction, landscaping, fishing, farming), uranium mining, radiology.
Soft tissue sarcomoas	Vinyl chloride, pesticides including chlorophenols and chlorophenoxy herbicides.	Farming, forestry workers.
Liver	Arsenic, vinyl chloride, organic solvents like trichloroethylene (TCE) and methylene chloride, polychlorinated biphynyls (PCBs), hepatitis B and C.	Petroleum and chemical industry workers, furniture refinishing, health care workers (due to needle stick accidents resulting in hepatitis B or C infection).
Bone	Ionizing radiation, radium.	Radium chemists, processors and dial painters.
Kidney	Arsenic, cadmium, lead, solvents including trichloroethylene (TCE) and tetrachloroethylene (PCE), coke oven emissions.	Laundry and dry-cleaning workers.
Brain	Metals including lead, arsenic and mercury. Solvents including benzene, toluene, xylene and methylene chloride, pesticides, oil refining, production of petrochemicals, synthetic rubber and polyvinyl chloride.	Chemists and workers in oil refineries, painters, wool and textile spinning, rubber industry workers, embalming.

Cancers Associated with Various Occupational Exposures		
CANCER	**SUBSTANCE OR PROCESS**	**WORKERS AT RISK**
Breast	Reactive chemicals like ethylene oxide, endocrine disruptors like certain pesticides and common plastics additives. Solvents including benzene, second-hand smoke, combustion by-products including polycyclic aromatic hydrocarbons (PAHs) and dioxin.	Industries using solvents including electronics and semiconductors, metal, lumbar, furniture, printing, chemical, and textile. Bartending.
Esophageal	Solvents including tetrachloroethylene (PCE), metal working fluids and mineral oils.	Dry-cleaning and dye-house workers, workers involved in grinding operations.
Cervical	Solvents like trichloroethylene (TCE) and tetrachloroethylene (PCE).	Dry cleaning.
Ovarian	Causal agent not identified, but may include solvents, mineral oils, PAHs, and printing inks and pigments.	Graphics and printing workers, hair dressing, beauticians.
Testicular	Polychlorinated biphenyls (PCBs) and hexachlorobenzene.	Agriculture, tanning, painting, mining, plastics, metal working, occupational use of hand-held radar.
Stomach	Lead, solvents including toluene, metal working fluids and mineral oils, asbestos.	Rubber industry workers. Coal, iron, lead, zinc and gold mining.

Cancers Associated with Various Occupational Exposures		
CANCER	**SUBSTANCE OR PROCESS**	**WORKERS AT RISK**
Pancreatic	Cadmium, nickel, methylene chloride, acrylamide.	Laundry and dry-cleaning workers.
Prostate	Some pesticides, metallic dusts, PAHs, cadmium, arsenic.	Metal working.
Rectal	Solvents including toluene, xylene. Metal working fluids and mineral oils.	Workers involved in grinding operations.

Common Household Products and Cancer Risk

"American consumers have no problem with carcinogens, but they will not purchase any product, including floor wax, that has fat in it."

—Dave Barry

In writing this book, the authors found several chemicals in their homes, despite their backgrounds in medicine, which needed to go. One bottle of hair spray found in a child's drawer contained a known human carcinogen that would be especially dangerous, since it was housed in an aerosol container. The label was too small to read until we pulled out a magnifying glass. But before we send our readers out to find expensive magnifying glasses usually reserved for use in the lab and for the blind, we recommend reading an excellent reference first. The National Institutes of Health hosts a household-product database listing many household products and their toxicity and carcinogenicity. For each product, it provides information about whether the chemical components have been listed under IARC, OSHA, or NTP as possibly causing cancer. Categories presented include auto, pesticides, personal care items, household cleaners, lawn products, pet care, and arts and crafts. This Web site can be accessed at http://householdproducts.nlm.nih.gov/products.htm.

Here is a list of chemical carcinogens and possible carcinogens you may have in your home and where they may be found:

- crystalline silica (cat litter, general cleaners, flea control products)
- trisodium nitrilotriacetate (laundry detergent)
- formaldehyde (car cleaners, furniture polish, paint, pressed wood furnishings, unwashed permanent press, wrinkle resistant or easy care clothing, preservative in many products)
- chlordane (home pesticides)
- nitrobenzene (furniture and floor polish, shoe polish)
- 1,4 dichlororbenzene (moth repellent)
- acid blue 9 (toilet bowl deodorizer)
- azo dyes (food additive)
- benzyl violet, also known as violet 2 or violet 6B (nail polish)
- naphthalene (moth repellent, toilet bowl deodorizer)
- paradichlorobenzene (moth repellent)
- oil of orange (household cleaners, spot removers)
- methylene chloride (spray paint, paint removers, shoe polish, adhesives and adhesive removers, glass frosting, water repellents)
- orange 3, red 49 (shoe polish)
- rotenone (flea control products)
- cobalt (artist oil paints)
- hexachlorobenzene (artist oil paints)
- aluminum silicate (paint)
- solvent dyes
- triethanolamine via reaction with nitrates (cleaning products)
- dibutyl phthalate (DBP) (nail polish)

- diethanolamine, triethanolamine via reaction with nitrates (moisturizers)
- polythylene glycol, bronopol, quaternium via release of formaldehyde (moisturizers, baby products)
- trichloroethylene (shoe polish, adhesives and adhesive removers, lubricating oils, leather care products, typewriter correction fluid)
- perchloroethylene or 1-1-1 trichloroethane (spot removers and carpet cleaners)

Many health-food stores, co-ops, and independent companies such as Melaleuca offer alternative household products based on the concerns we have addressed. In Table 4-4 we list some "old-fashioned," yet time-tested household staples that can be substituted for commercial products as well.

Table 4-4. Alternatives to Common Household Products

Alternatives to Common Household Products	
Household Product	**Alternative**
Adhesive removers	Soak item with decals or residual glue in white vinegar.
Air fresheners	Open windows; simmer water with lemon slices or a mixture of cinnamon and cloves on the stove; use baking soda for carpet odors and keep an open box in the refrigerator; bowls of potpourri; houseplants can help with odors and also eliminate toxins such as formaldehyde; add ½ cup of borax to the bottom of garbage cans.
All-purpose cleaner	Use a 50:50 solution of water and white vinegar, or try a solution of 4 tbsp of baking soda in one quart of water.
Aluminum	Clean with a solution of one-quart hot water and 2 tbsp cream of tarter; lemon juice can remove stains on aluminum.
Ant repellent	Seal areas where ants enter; use cinnamon, dried mint, borax, or red chili peppers at entry points.

Alternatives to Common Household Products	
Household Product	**Alternative**
Brass cleaner	Clean with Worcestershire sauce, a soft cloth dipped in a lemon juice and baking soda solution, or try equal parts vinegar, salt, and flour; always rinse well to avoid corrosion.
Carpet deodorizer	Spread baking soda on carpeting one half hour before vacuuming.
Chemical mouse killers	Sticky traps and mousetraps; cats as pets.
Chemical weed killers	Boiling water; hand-pulling weeds; landscaping to minimize weeds; learn to tolerate a few weeds; mulch.
Chrome	Clean with apple cider vinegar.
Commercial cleaning products	Several alternative cleaners are available at your local health food store or co-op.
Commercial cleansers	Baking soda.
Copper cleaner	Boil in water with one cup of vinegar and 1 tbsp salt.
Disinfectants	Use plain isopropyl alcohol (keep out of reach of children).
Drain cleaners	A plunger or plumber's snake; add ½-cup baking soda and ½-cup vinegar to the drain and cover, allowing the chemical reaction to clean the drain. After 15 minutes, add boiling water. Do not use this if you have used a commercial drain cleaner.
Fabric bleach	Add a small amount of borax (cautiously, since this can be toxic) to the wash cycle; apply lemon juice to stains and place in the sun.
Fabric softeners	Add a cup of baking soda to the wash to soften and decrease static cling, or add ½ to one cup of white vinegar to the rinse cycle.
Fabric starch	Plain cornstarch.

Alternatives to Common Household Products	
Household Product	**Alternative**
Flea products	Flea combs; frequent vacuuming; wash your pet and pet bedding often; try alternative products when necessary.
Furniture polish	Mix 1 tsp of lemon juice with a pint of olive or mineral oil.
Garden insecticides	Ladybugs (available at several nurseries); clean the leaves of indoor houseplants with water and a soft cloth.
Laundry detergent	Natural soap flakes.
Lawn pesticides and fertilizers	Organic fertilizer or compost; aerate your lawn, and mow high and often; leave clippings on the lawn.
Linoleum floor cleaner	Mix 1 cup of vinegar in 2 gallons of warm water.
Lubricants such as WD-40 (R)	Alternative lubricants can be purchased at your health food store; olive oil.
Mosquito repellent	Bug lights; citronella candles; protective clothing; avoiding dusk; sweet basil near your deck or patio.
Mothballs	Cedar planks; store wools in airtight containers; placing items in the dryer for a short while can kill moth eggs.
Oven cleaner	Heat (self-cleaning ovens); baking soda; moist cloth; steel wool; for stubborn residue, apply baking soda and sprinkle with water until it is moist. Continue to keep the area moist for twelve hours and then scrub; Arm and Hammer® oven cleaner is considered safe.
Silver polish	Place silver in a pan of boiling water lined with aluminum foil, add 1 tsp of salt and 1 tsp of baking soda.
Window cleaner	Fill a spray bottle with water and add 1 tbsp lemon juice and 4 tbsp vinegar; clean windows early or late in the day when the sun is lower to avoid streaking.
Wood floor cleaner	A solution of one to one vinegar and oil, and polish.

Practical Points

- ❑ Have your home tested for radon.
- ❑ Open windows and doors frequently to bring fresh air into your home.
- ❑ Practice caution with any chemical you use. Use gloves, a proper mask, leave products in their original containers, and always dispose of hazardous materials safely.
- ❑ Wash clothes and linens that are "permanent press," "wrinkle resistant," or easy care prior to wearing or sleeping.
- ❑ Protect yourself from the sun with a hat, umbrella, and protective clothing. Avoid being in the sun between 11 a.m. and 3 p.m. Use sunscreen to prevent sunburns. If you can find the new sunscreen available which also covers UVA rays, discard your old lotions, and use the newer one containing Mexoryl™SX instead.
- ❑ Invest in "healthy" houseplants to clean your indoor air.
- ❑ If you have well water, have it tested.
- ❑ Purchase a water filter, preferably a reverse osmosis system, for the water you drink and cook with.
- ❑ Minimize use of home and garden pesticides.
- ❑ Avoid dry-cleaning clothes; consider wet-cleaning as an alternative.
- ❑ Avoid commercial air fresheners.

Resources and Further Online Information

Household Products Database

www.householdproducts.nlm.nih.gov/products.htm

This database from the National Institutes of Health and the National Library of Medicine provides information on the health effects, carcinogenicity, and handling suggestions for many products. Ingredients are listed that are not frequently found on labels. Categories include: auto products, home maintenance, inside-the-home products, pesticides, landscape/yard, personal care, pet care, and arts and crafts.

U.S. EPA. Radon

www.epa.gov/radon/

This Web site addresses the health risks, and answers questions individuals may have about radon exposure. It also provides links for further information regarding testing for radon levels, and fixing elevated levels. Links are available for information based on your state of residence. Those that are building a new home can, in addition learn about radon-resistant new construction. The EPA can also be contacted at 1-800-SOS-RADON.

Additional information on radon can be obtained by contacting The National Safety Council at 1-800-767-7326 or The National Radon Fix-it-up Program at 1-800-644-6699.

Discounted radon test kits can be purchased through the National Radon Helpline at 1-800-557-2366.

U.S. EPA. SunWise Program

www.epa.gov/sunwise/uvindex.html

Based on zip code or city, you can obtain the UV index and UV index forecast for your location.

CTIA The Wireless Foundation

www.donateaphone.com

This site provides information on how to recycle old cell phones, as well general information on cell phone safety and etiquette.

U.S. EPA. Clean Burning Woodstoves and Fireplaces
www.epa.gov/woodstoves/index.html

The EPA provides this Web site that has helpful information for those with woodstoves and conventional fireplaces. A section titled "Healthier Home, Cleaner Environment" discusses why wood smoke can be harmful to your health. For those interested in fireplace inserts and other options, information about these is available as well.

U.S. EPA. Design for the Environment. Garment and Textile Care Program. The Cleaner Guide. A List of Professional Cleaners Offering Professional Wetcleaning or Liquid Carbon Dioxide Cleaning Processes
www.epa.gov/dfe/pubs/garment/gcrg/cleanquide.pdf

This EPA site provides addresses for wet cleaners, listed by state.

U.S. EPA. Ground Water and Drinking Water
www.epa.gov/safewater/links.html

This site contains general information about what you need to know about your drinking water, and offers links to water protection programs by state. For general information the EPA also provides a safe drinking water hotline at 1-800-426-4791.

U.S. EPA. Pesticides: Topical and Chemical Fact Sheets
www.epa.gov/pesticides/factsheets/alpha_fs.htm

This web site provides extensive information on specific pesticides, as well as a wealth of safety information. Links are provided covering issues ranging from pesticide use in the home to mosquito control.

The National Pesticide Information Center (NPIC)
1-800-858-7378

The NPIC provides information about pesticide products and toxicity.

U.S. EPA. Citizen's Guide to Pest Control and Pesticide Safety
www.epa.gov/OPPTpubs/Cit_Guide/citguide.pdf

The EPA citizen's guide is a must for anyone who is struggling with pests in their home environment. This site provides information on preventing pests, chemical and non-chemical means for eliminating pests, ways to reduce your exposure when others use pesticides, and even information on how to choose a pest control company when needed.

Environmental Working Group. Ten safety steps to reduce your family's exposure to arsenic from arsenic treated wood
www.ewg.org/issues/arsenic/10tips.php

The Environmental Working Group (EWG) understands that despite their recommendation to replace structures built from arsenic treated wood, this is prohibitively expensive for many families. In response, they offer many helpful tips to reduce an individual's exposure to arsenic from existing structures. If you would like to test for arsenic in your current structures or test the soil beneath them, information on arsenic test kits can be obtained at www.ewg.org/reports/poisonwoodrivals/orderform.php.

U.S. EPA. Asbestos
www.epa.gov/asbestos/

The EPA Website about asbestos covers many topics including asbestos in the home. If you need information on removal or remodeling, you can also contact the EPA's TSCA assistance line at 1-202-5554-1414.

National Institute of Occupational Safety and Health (NIOSH). Chemical Safety
www.cdc.gov/niosh/topics/chemical-safety

NIOSH provides multiple databases regarding occupational chemical safety, and also has a toll free number for questions about occupational exposures at 1-800-356-4674.

OSHA has a 24-hour access line to report unsafe work practices at 1-800-321-6742.

U.S. EPA. Toxics Release Inventory (TRI) Program
www.epa.gov/tri

This site provides information regarding toxic chemical releases by industry in your neighborhood.

U.S. EPA. Indoor Air Quality (IAQ). An Introduction to Indoor Air Quality
www.epa.gov/iaq/ia-intro.html

On this site the EPA lists pollutants and sources of indoor air pollution you may have in your home with information on how to improve your indoor air quality based on specific pollutants.

Office of Environmental Health Hazard Assessment (OEHHA). Proposition 65
www.oehha.ca.gov/prop65.html

Proposition 65, the Safe Water and Toxic Enforcement Act of 1986, requires the

Governor of California to publish yearly a list of chemicals known to cause cancer. Substances currently felt to carry a risk for the development of cancer in individuals exposed to them are listed on this site.

International Agency for Research on Cancer (IARC)
www.iarc.fr/

IARC provides information on substances felt to be carcinogenic to humans.

National Toxicology Program
http://ntp.niehs.nib.gov/index.cfm?objectid=72016262-BDB7-CEBA-FA60E922B182540

The NTP has two lists, known carcinogens, and reasonably anticipated to be carcinogens, that can be accessed online though this Web site. Copies can also be ordered by mail at Central Data Management (CDM), MD-EC-03, NIEHS, P.O. Box 12233 Research Triangle Park, NC 27709. A request can also be faxed to NTP at 1-919-541-3687.

National Institute for Occupational Safety and Health (NIOSH). NIOSH Carcinogen List
www.cdc.gov/niosh/npotocca.htm

This site provides a list of substances which NIOSH believes are potential occupational carcinogens.

Whole Foods Market
www.wholefoods.com

Whole Foods Market has many locations nationwide, and offers alternative household products that have been examined for safety.

Fresh and Natural Foods (Minnesota and Wisconsin only)
www.freshandnaturalfoods.com

This Web site provides information on store locations, and carries a line of healthy alternative household products.

The WEDGE Natural Foods Co-op (Minnesota only)
www.wedge.coop/

The Wedge carries alternative household products in addition to its selection of healthy food.

Good Earth Natural Foods (California only)
www.goodearthnaturalfoods.net

Good Earth Natural Foods carries household products that can be used as an alternative to many commercial products.

Sun Organic Farm
www.sunorganicfarm.com

Sun Organic Farm is an online health food store that offers delivery of organic and natural products to your door. A free organic food and product catalogue can be obtained by calling them toll free at 1-888-269-9888.

Seventh Generation
www.seventhgen.com

Seventh Generation products were designed as safer alternatives to many commercial household products. This Web site provides general information on household hazards. Locations of stores in your area that carry these products can be found by entering your zip code.

Melaleuca
www.melaleuca.com

Melaleuca offers alternative personal care and household products at wholesale prices. For information on obtaining these products you can email todayshealth.wellness@yahoo.com.

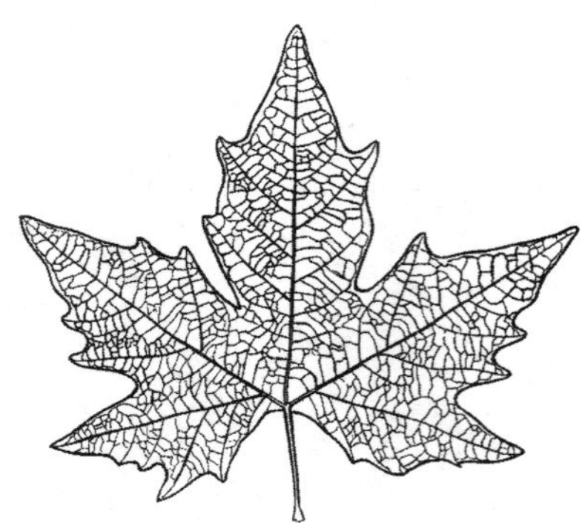

Chapter Five

Infection and Cancer Prevention

"Anyone could experience this very severe, life-threatening illness."

—Dr. Michael Osterholm

Despite progress unrivaled anywhere else in medicine over the last 100 years, microorganisms, including viruses, bacteria, and parasites, account for approximately 10 percent of cancers diagnosed in the United States and 25 percent of cases worldwide. Infectious diseases causing or predisposing those who contract them to cancer are of particular interest since great strides have been made in our ability to control disease caused by microscopic menaces. A century ago, children frequently died from infections that have now become only nuisances requiring a day off school and a prescription of antibiotics. Parents fret more about what they will do about childcare for a day or about who will take a day off work than they do about whether or not they will lose a child. Many previously fatal and disabling infectious diseases are almost unheard of due to the advent of widespread vaccination.

Smallpox has been eradicated worldwide (hopefully); diphtheria is not a common household word. Most people have not heard of anyone who has died from tetanus. Mothers-to-be do not go through pregnancy fearing they will develop German measles (Rubella) and have a deformed baby. The introduction of vaccines and antibiotics has created a world where we have forgotten or may never hear of the devastation from those miniature bugs that have proved so lethal in the past. The authors have a grandmother who worked with Sister Kinney during the polio epidemic. Her stories have not been forgotten.

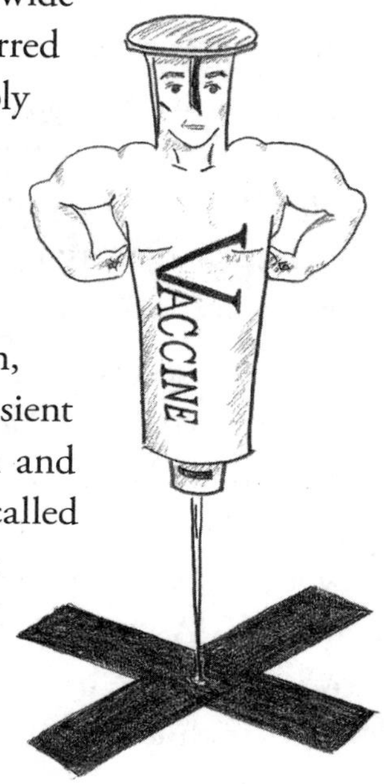

In 1967, the World Health Organization started a worldwide campaign to eradicate smallpox. The last reported case occurred in Somalia in 1977, and on May 8, 1980, the World Assembly declared the world free from smallpox. This occurred in the days before Internet mail and electronic medical records. How wonderful it would be if we could make similar strides with cancer, so that, a few generations from now, some previously common cancers would be nearly forgotten, and those that manage to show their face would only be transient setbacks. How thankful we would be if our grandchildren and great-grandchildren did not know there was an infection called hepatitis B that could cause cancer, as well as significant morbidity and mortality, except through their studies to answer questions on honors history tests. Imagine the celebration if Pap smears were deemed an archaic procedure no longer needed because the virus that caused cervical cancer had been eradicated, or at least prevented by vaccination? Speculums could be placed in museums next to fifteenth-century relics of torture! Perhaps with the widespread immunization of all children for hepatitis B, and the recent approval of the HPV vaccine, we may witness the primary prevention of cancer through vaccination (albeit a small percentage of cases) in our lifetime!

Before we get too lofty in our visions, we need to take off our blinders and recall that, while a few bad bugs from the past have been placed behind bars, previously unknown enemies have entered the picture, armed with even greater artillery. Instead of confronting smallpox, with its casualty rate of 25 percent, we have met HIV (AIDS), a force that kills any civilian it encounters with 100 percent accuracy. In the United States, we have seen this terrorist overtake and control many Americans, infecting and ruling the lives of at least 400,000 people currently alive who grew up saying the Pledge of Allegiance. In parts of Africa, those controlled by the terrorist may soon outnumber those who are still free. This terrorist, unlike smallpox, which made its kill quickly or fled, allows its victims to suffer for lengthy periods, often with cancers it causes, and it never leaves without finishing the act. Unlike smallpox, HIV/AIDS does not sit still long enough for scientists to develop anti-miniscule warfare: a vaccine is not yet available. And unlike smallpox, which has cousins that attack cows and monkeys, HIV has brothers and sisters in hiding that would happily visit humans; these include two that we have seen for awhile and two that just emerged in 2005 about which we know little. Before we begin to look at infectious causes of cancer as "easy" causes to deal with, we need to make it clear that emerging infectious diseases and threats of bioterrorism could change our concept of cancer prevention in a heartbeat.

There seems to be less awareness of the role infections play in predisposing individuals to cancer relative to other causes. Many people are aware that smoked and pickled foods are correlated with stomach cancer; fewer appear to be aware that *H. pylori*, the bacteria that causes most ulcers, is the leading cause of stomach cancer worldwide. Many understand a trip to Mexico could be ruined if they picked up hepatitis A, but fewer have heard that 80 percent of liver cancer throughout the world is caused by hepatitis B, even after they have carefully written down the dates of their childrens' hepatitis B shots on school forms.

This is also an area laden heavily with emotion. With the HPV vaccine now approved, advocacy groups are addressing the possible impact. Rather than being celebrated as a way to prevent perhaps 70 percent of cases of cervical cancer, this vaccine generates the fear that being vaccinated will give young girls permission to have sex. Instead of reminding ourselves that the HPV vaccine does not prevent pregnancy, AIDS, and a host of other sexually transmitted diseases, we are reduced to picturing our young, perfect children becoming sexually active too early. There is also a general distrust of the pharmaceutical industry, which is sometimes viewed as being in business for cold hard cash rather than for the prevention of disease.

Prevention may have been easier in the past. When the polio vaccine became available, the public cheered. Most people knew of, or had heard of, someone whose life was forever changed from the infection. We were not bombarded by emails, Internet pop-ups, and blogs discussing the disadvantages or possible evils associated with vaccines. The oral polio vaccine was not without side effects, and the authors are sincerely saddened for those who did have the rare side effects. We know that those who suffered could have been our children as well, and wish to reassure the readers that we understand statistics: success rates become somehow meaningless if you happen to be the "case" that had a "side effect." Yet many people were spared paralysis, disability, and death. Statistically, vaccination for polio was a great success.

Prevention, or at least containment of infectious disease, may have been easier in days gone by as well. During the polio epidemic, families left the city during the summer and fled to the country to avoid exposure. With our lust now for international and adventure travel, business enterprises that span the globe, and in a time when three commercial flights can take us nearly anywhere in the world, we are exposed to and can carry more germs to the ends of the earth than our counterparts a few generations back could fathom. Keeping this in mind, it is important to be aware of some infections not typically found in the United States as well as those endemic to our country: several that can predispose a person to developing cancer.

In addition to the well-known infectious symptoms they create, microorganisms can cause cancer to develop in several ways. With oncoviruses (cancer causing viruses) the virus enters cells and can cause cancer by directly affecting DNA. In other cases, such as with HIV, the virus damages the immune system, so the individual is unable to fight off the cancer cells that develop periodically in all of us. In many cases, such as with hepatitis B and C, *H. pylori*, HPV and parasitic infections, the organism creates chronic inflammation, leading to increased cell division for repair, which raises the risk for mutations that lead to cancer. In some cases, like EBV (mono), we remain clueless about why the virus predisposes a person to develop cancer and question why it is more significant if the infection starts in adolescence than in childhood, since in both instances the virus is usually "carried" for life.

Hepatitis B

Hepatitis B was the only infectious cause of cancer preventable by vaccination until June of 2006, when the HPV vaccine was approved. While progression to liver cancer occurs in only a small percentage of people who develop infection with hepatitis B, it is estimated that 80 percent of liver cancer worldwide is associated with chronic hepatitis B infection. In the United States 15 percent of liver cancer is due to hepatitis B, with most of the remaining cases caused by hepatitis C infection and cirrhosis from alcohol abuse. Studies have concluded that widespread immunization for hepatitis B **can** reduce cancer. Universal childhood immunization against hepatitis B in Taiwan decreased the incidence of liver cancer in children by 49 percent between 1981 and 1994 (Chang, 1997). Other studies have shown a decreased incidence of liver cancer in adults immunized as well.

Hepatitis B is a virus that can be transmitted through blood products and sexual contact, but in many cases the source of transmission is unknown. Hepatitis B, which is one-hundred times more contagious than HIV, can be transmitted even by sharing a toothbrush! While risk factors for hepatitis B include intravenous drug abuse, high-risk sexual behavior, and occupational exposure to blood products, in over half of cases a known source of exposure or high-risk behavior is not present. Despite recommendations for adults in high-risk groups to receive the vaccine, the incidence of hepatitis B in the Unites States has increased. Routine vaccination for hepatitis B is now recommended for all children and adolescents in the United States.

People who acquire an infection with hepatitis B early in life are much more likely to carry the disease, and therefore spread it to those around them. Developing the infection later in life is more likely to result in severe disease and possibly death, but less likely to result in a chronic carrier state, due to differences in how the immune system handles the virus. Routine hepatitis B testing of pregnant women in the United States and prophylactic treatment of babies born to infected mothers, in addition to vaccinating children, should reduce this risk substantially. For those who carry hepatitis B, effective treatment is now available that may lower the risk of developing liver cancer. Hepatitis B carriers should also avoid substances that can cause liver damage, such as alcohol, and should be immunized against hepatitis A.

HEPATITIS C

"We stand at the precipice of a grave threat to our public health…It affects people from all walks of life, in every state, in every country. And unless we do something about it soon, it will kill more people than AIDS."

—C. Everett Koop, Former U.S. Surgeon General, on hepatitis C

Hepatitis C, a virus first identified in 1989, is currently the leading cause of liver cancer in the United States and the most common reason for liver transplantation. Infection with hepatitis C also significantly increases the incidence of non-Hodgkin's lymphoma and multiple myeloma. Until 1989, physicians were aware that some patients developed hepatitis after a blood transfusion not attributable to either hepatitis A or B. Hepatitis C (HCV) was simply known as nonA-nonB hepatitis and no test was available to screen for this disease. Understanding of this infection has come a long way in the last decade or so. The causative agent was isolated, and with that, it became possible to screen blood products for the virus. With the virus identified, it also became possible to test for virus levels in the body and subsequently develop treatments to clear the infection. Hepatitis C is now a treatable disease in many cases.

Even though infection with HCV is much more common than HIV, with an estimated 1.8 percent of the population having been infected, public awareness has lagged behind. The Institute of Medicine has labeled HCV as an emerging infectious disease and the CDC predicts that deaths secondary to HCV will double or triple in the next fifteen to twenty years. Although the infection rate has declined with the screening of blood products, the long latency period between onset of infection and progression to disease (ten to forty years) means there are many people infected who have not yet manifested symptoms. A significant percentage of those who carry the disease are unaware of what is brewing in their liver.

Hepatitis C is transmitted in a way similar to hepatitis B, through blood-to-blood contact. This is in contrast to hepatitis A, which is spread by contaminated food and water. Until July of 1989, it was not possible to screen for HCV and many people contracted the infection through blood transfusions. Currently the most common mode of transmission is through IV drug abuse. Like hepatitis B, hepatitis C can be transmitted sexually; through needle sticks; sharing razors, toothbrushes, nail clippers; body piercing, and tattooing. Hepatitis C can also be transferred from a mother to a child during pregnancy and childbirth, but this is much less common than with hepatitis B. Thirty percent of the time it is unknown how the infection was acquired.

Many people who carry the disease have not been tested, and 80 percent of the time there are no symptoms until advanced liver disease sets in. When symptoms occur, they include fatigue, flu-like symptoms, abdominal pain, and jaundice. Treatment strategies have improved remarkably and, depending on the strain, cure rates with a combination of interferon and an anti-viral medication are around 50 percent. A few alternative remedies are also showing promise. If someone is diagnosed with HCV, they should avoid alcohol and be immunized against hepatitis A and B to avoid further damage to the liver. There is not a vaccine available for hepatitis C at this time.

In light of this information, who should be screened? The CDC recommends the following people have a blood test to screen for hepatitis C:

- persons who have ever injected illegal drugs, including those who injected once or a few times many years ago
- persons who were treated for clotting problems with a blood product made before 1987, when more advanced methods for manufacturing the products were developed
- persons who were notified that they received blood from a donor who later tested positive for hepatitis C
- persons who received a blood transfusion or solid organ transplant before July 1992, when better testing of blood donors became available
- long-term hemodialysis patients
- persons who have signs or symptoms of liver disease (e.g., abnormal liver enzyme tests)
- healthcare workers after exposures (e.g., needle sticks or splashes to the eye) to HVC-positive blood on the job

- children born to HCV-positive women

Source: CDC. Viral hepatitis C. Who should get tested for hepatitis C. Accessible at www.cdc.gov/ncidod/diseases/hepatitis/c/faq.htm#7a.

HIV/AIDS

HIV, the virus that causes AIDS, is a well-known cause of many cancers, especially Kaposi's sarcoma and lymphomas. HIV inflicts its harm by progressively damaging the immune system, disabling the body's natural cancer-fighting cells, leaving cancer cells that occur in all of us unchecked to grow out of control, and leaving the body susceptible to bacteria that ordinarily do not cause infections. The weakened immune system of AIDS patients also lets carcinogenic viruses, such as hepatitis B and C, Kaposi's sarcoma herpes virus/human herpes virus 8, and HPV, proliferate. Most patients succumb from these infections or cancers. Since information about HIV has been much more widely published than information about other infectious causes of cancer, we refer those who are interested to a few excellent sources of information listed in the resources at the end of this chapter.

Epstein Barr Virus/Infectious Mononucleosis

Commonly known simply as "mono" in the United States, infection with the Epstein-Barr virus (EBV) has caused more problems than trying to deal with a teenager sleeping twenty hours a day and missing school. This virus was discovered forty years ago as the culprit that causes the symptoms of infectious mononucleosis, the dreaded disease that wreaks havoc on many a high school student's GPA. It was also the first virus known to cause cancer through its actions on the body.

Worldwide, approximately 90 percent of people have been infected with EBV. Most infections occur in early childhood through contact with the saliva of friends or caretakers, hence its pseudonym the "kissing disease," and are usually asymptomatic. Clinical illness is usually seen only when the primary infection is delayed until the teen years or later in life, due to the bodies more aggressive immune response at this stage. One third to one-half of teens who acquire the virus develop the classic syndrome, infectious mononucleosis. Once the EB virus infects the body, it persists for life, living in B-lymphocytes (a type of white blood cell).

The Epstein-Barr virus has long been known as the cause of Burkett's lymphoma, a cancer much more common in sub-Saharan Africa than elsewhere, and nasopharyngeal cancer. Recent studies have implicated EBV in several other cancer types, and the International Association for Research on Cancer (IARC) has now classified EBV as a class 1 carcinogen. Cancers in which EBV appears to play a role include Burkett's lymphoma, nasopharyngeal carcinoma, Hodgkin's disease, non-Hodgkin's lymphoma, certain cancers in immunosuppressed individuals, and gastric cancer, and it may possibly be a cofactor in breast cancer.

Hodgkin's disease is one of the most common cancers in teens and young adults in the United States. EBV is estimated to be involved in the development of over 40 percent of cases of Hodgkin's disease worldwide, and is found in the cancer cells of those people in the U.S. with Hodgkin's disease half of the time. The average time between mononucleosis and the development of Hodgkin's disease is roughly two years, and approximately one out of a thousand people diagnosed with mono develop this cancer. Even though the Epstein-Barr virus persists in the body for life, developing the infection later in life, such as during the teen years, plays a greater role in the development of Hodgkin's disease and gastric cancer than acquiring the infection earlier.

An understanding of timing may offer some assistance, at least concerning primary prevention. While we know little about who is predisposed to developing cancer following a bout of infectious mononucleosis, we do not have to wait to take some action. If you or someone in your family has been diagnosed with mono, we would recommend following closely the other principles in this book, especially the nutrition recommendations. If you struggle maintaining a healthy diet, consider employing a nutritionist to help you. Carefully review lifestyle issues for anything you can change to otherwise lower your risk.

Human Papillomavirus (HPV)

As if the fear of pregnancy, syphilis, and AIDS were not enough, we now know that sexually transmitted infection with the human papillomavirus causes nearly all cases of cervical cancer, roughly 25 percent of oral cancers, and is associated with anal, penile, and vaginal cancer. To confuse things further, of the roughly 200 strains of HPV, at least one of which is present in an estimated 75 percent of sexually active adults, infection with only a few strains can progress to cancer. Since discussion concerning HPV covers several dimensions of prevention, both primary and secondary, in addition to being emotionally laden and confusing, we will expand on this in some depth. Primary prevention can be practiced by engaging in safe sex, being immunized against the virus, and by incorporating dietary changes that have been shown to help clear the infection and consequently lower the risk of cancer if you develop the infection. Secondary prevention through regular screening with Pap smears allows for early detection and treatment of cervical dysplasia, preventing its progressing to cancer.

As noted above, HPV comprises a large group of viruses that are extremely common. Many of these are entirely asymptomatic. Some of these cause genital warts in both men and women. A few strains, namely HPV 16 and HPV 18, as well as HPV 31, 33, 35, 39, 45, 51, 52, 56, 58, 59, 68, 69 and possibly others, are considered the cancer causing strains, with HPV 16 estimated to cause around 50 percent and HPV 58 24 percent of cervical cancers. These strains of HPV infect the uterine cervix, causing inflammation that sometimes results in dysplasia (abnormal changes which can be a precursor to cancer) and cancer. Men infected with these strains do not have any symptoms, with the extremely rare exception of penile cancer. Not all infections with cancer-causing strains of HPV result in disease, and in fact, the majority of infections resolve on their own. Factors that increase the odds of the infection lingering and proceeding to dysplasia and possibly cancer include smoking, having given birth to several children, and having a damaged immune system.

Since the majority of high-risk HPV infections are asymptomatic (people do not have any symptoms of an illness) until they progress to disease, it is difficult to know who may carry these strains. Men and women considering physical relationships with new partners can ask each other if they have had, or have been sexually active with anyone who has had, an abnormal Pap smear, history of dysplasia, cervical cancer, or has been told they carry high-risk forms of HPV. The use of condoms, if this is the case, decreases the risk of transmission but does not eliminate it.

Being uncircumcised increases the risk of contracting penile HPV infection and in the case of men with multiple sexual partners, it increases the risk of cervical cancer in their female partners (Castellsague, 2002). Researchers who published this information in *The New England Journal of Medicine* were met with strong opposition and inspired editorials about ethics and male sexual issues. This information does **not** call for global circumcision. Nor should it be the cause for needless debate between men rallying for the rights to their foreskin and women wishing to protect themselves from cancer. This information should simply enable uncircumcised men who choose to have multiple partners to be knowledgeable enough to inform someone they are with of the risk, advise them to see a healthcare provider for regular exams, and discuss precautions such as the use of condoms. Likewise, women who are with uncircumcised men outside of committed relationships and who know the risks can insist on the use of condoms.

A vaccine to prevent infection with several strains of HPV has now been released. In clinical trials, the vaccine has been shown to prevent infection with HPV 16 and HPV 18 100 percent of the time with protection still present after four to five years (Harper, 2006). These two strains of HPV cause 70 percent of cases of cervical cancer in the United States. It is important to note that the vaccine does not prevent cancer per se. It prevents the infection that causes inflammation that can lead to cancer, and therefore should be given prior to women becoming sexually active if possible.

Secondary prevention through widespread cervical screening using Pap smears has dramatically reduced the progression of HPV-induced dysplasia on to cancer in the United States. Worldwide, cervical cancer is the second most common cancer in women, but only the eighth most common cancer in women in the U.S. A recent study published in *Lancet* revealed evidence that cervical screening has prevented an epidemic that would have killed one in sixty-five British women born since 1950

(Peto, 2004). In most cases, though not all, there is a significant period between infection with the virus and development of cervical cancer and therefore yearly screening has been very effective.

Abnormal Pap smears can occur for many reasons, only one of which is the presence of HPV. When a Pap smear is abnormal, it is now customary to check for HPV. The results are then evaluated based on whether or not the strains are high risk or low risk. Depending on the results of the Pap smear, most people with low-risk strains will not require further testing other than a repeat Pap smear in one year. For those people found to have one or more high-risk strains, further testing with colposcopy and possibly biopsies is indicated.

While it is clear that HPV is the causative agent of most cases of cervical cancer, it is currently felt to be responsible for roughly 25 percent of oral cancers as well (Scully, 2002). Significantly higher levels of the cancer-causing HPV viruses, especially HPV 16, are found in the mouths of patients with oral cancer than in those without oral cancer. Those patients with positive HPV 16 are unlikely to fit the stereotypical patient with oral cancer, in that the incidence of smoking and drinking alcohol in this group is low. Thankfully, the prognosis for the HPV group appears to be much better. The idea that HPV is implicated in the development of oral cancers is recent, and the authors were unable to find any specific screening recommendations based on these findings. If you happen to have been diagnosed with high-risk HPV, have had abnormal Pap smears requiring follow-up, or, for men, have had a partner experience this, we recommend monthly, oral self-exams and scheduling regular dental exams. Many dentists routinely screen for oral cancer now during preventive health visits.

Most infections with HPV resolve without progressing to dysplasia and cancer. For those diagnosed with HPV, studies have shown a diet high in vegetables correlates with a resolution of the infection. Increased dietary intake of lutein/zeaxanthin, beta-cryptoxanthin, vitamin C, vitamin A, lycopene, and papaya lower the risk of persistent HPV and therefore the potential for cancer to develop (Sedjo, 2002). Good sources of these include:

- Lutein/zeaxanthin – spinach, kale, turnips, mustard and collard greens
- Beta-cryptoxanthin – pumpkins, red peppers, papayas, tangerines

- Vitamin C – orange juice, red peppers, grapefruit juice, peaches
- Vitamin A – turkey, carrot juice, pumpkins, sweet potatoes, carrots, spinach
- Lycopene – tomato products, especially sauces
- Papaya – fresh papaya, papaya nectar

In one study, the use of tampons decreased the rate of HPV clearance (Richardson, 2005). Women diagnosed with high-risk strains of HPV may want to consider using sanitary napkins as an alternative.

Human T Cell Lymphotropic Virus (HTLV-1)

Human T cell lymphotropic virus (HTLV) is a retrovirus, a class of viruses that includes viruses such as HIV. Infection is uncommon in the United States, but it is estimated that 15 to 20 million people have been infected with HTLV-1 worldwide. Of those infected, roughly two to five percent will develop adult T cell leukemia/lymphoma (ATLL). HTLV-1 clusters in certain areas of the world and is most commonly found in Japan, the Caribbean, parts of South America, Papua New Guinea, and central and west Africa. HTLV-1 is transmitted through blood, sexually, and from mother to infant primarily via breast-feeding. In Japan, women are tested when pregnant and, if positive, are advised not to breastfeed, since transition of the virus through breast milk is a major route of transmission in high prevalence areas. HTLV-2 causes some noncancerous symptoms seen with HTLV-1 and is found in Native Americans, South American Indians, and in some parts of the Caribbean. Very recently, two new retroviruses, HTLV-3 and HTLV-4 appeared in Cameroon. Though not yet linked to any disease, they are related to HIV and HTLV-1, which have caused major devastation. It is felt that these infections were transmitted to humans from monkeys through bites and scratches while the humans were hunting. If these viruses prove to carry any of the characteristics of their closely related brothers, discouraging those who hunt for monkeys and apes for food may become a primary prevention measure.

SCHISTOSOMIASIS AND LIVER FLUKES

Bladder cancer, secondary to the infectious disease schistosomiasis, also known as bilharzia, is the leading cause of death of men between the ages of twenty and forty-four in Egypt. In some regions of Africa, infection with the schistosome parasite is associated with a rate of bladder cancer thirty-two times that of the rate in the United States. Although it is estimated that only 400,000 people in the United States, primarily immigrants and people who have traveled to endemic regions, are infected, the toll worldwide is over 200,000 million people. Africa, Asia, and South America are the regions most affected. Schistosoma flatworms (flukes) live in snails in contaminated fresh water. When people swim or wade in contaminated water, the parasites penetrate through unbroken skin, mature into larva, and become the adult worms that cause chronic infection in the bladder, intestines, and other locations, depending on the type of flatworm. This chronic infection creates inflammation, which in turn causes increased cell division during repair, increasing the risk of mutations that can lead to cancer.

Since even brief exposure can result in infection, avoid swimming or wading in fresh water in regions where Shistosomiasis occurs. Boiling water for one minute prior to drinking will kill the parasite. Heating bath water to 122° F before bathing is recommended as well. Schistosomiasis is not found in the ocean, and chlorine-treated swimming pools are considered safe.

Initial infection with Schistosomiasis is often asymptomatic but can be accompanied by a rash or flu-like symptoms (Katayama Fever), and occasionally neurological symptoms. If you have traveled to a high-risk region, consider being tested for infection. Urine and stool tests are available, but most accurate is a blood test available through the CDC. Safe and effective treatment is available.

The CDC lists the following locations where Schistosomiasis is commonly found:

- South America: including Brazil, Suriname, Venezuela
- Caribbean: Antigua, Dominican Republic, Guadeloupe, Martinique, Montserrat, Saint Lucia (risk is low)
- The Middle East: Iran, Iraq, Saudi Arabia, Syrian Arab Republic, Yemen

- Southern China
- Southeast Asia: Philippines, Laos, Cambodia, Japan, central Indonesia, Mekong delta
- Africa: Lake Malawi, the Nile River valley in Egypt

If you travel, it is a good idea to check for information that is as recent as possible. In some regions, schistosomiasis has been eliminated, whereas in others it is increasing. Up-to-date information on endemic infections based on region is available at the CDC's Web site at www.cdc.gov/travel/.

Liver flukes, which are found primarily in East Asia, are a significant cause of bile duct cancer (cholangiocarcinoma), a cancer rare in the United States. In northeast Thailand, the incidence of bile duct cancer is forty times higher than the incidence found outside of Thailand. Liver flukes are contracted by eating raw or undercooked freshwater fish that have been contaminated by the parasite. After being ingested, the mature flukes chronically infect the pancreas and gall bladder. Most infections are asymptomatic.

Stool and blood tests, as well as radiological procedures, can diagnose most infections, and effective treatment is available. When traveling in this region, avoid freshwater fish that are not cooked thoroughly.

H. Pylori

Epidemiological evidence suggests that 60-90 percent of gastric (stomach) cancers are attributable to infection with *Helicobacter pylori (H. pylori)*, a ubiquitous bacterium discovered in 1982. *H. pylori* infects the lining of the stomach, causing inflammation, ulcers, and gastritis. Infection with these bacteria is responsible for 90 percent of duodenal and 80 percent of gastric ulcers, collectively accounting for more than a million hospitalizations annually, and raises the risk of developing gastric cancer two to sixfold. While gastric cancer has been declining in the United States since the 1930s, it remains the fourth most common form of cancer worldwide.

Knowing the causative agent for the majority of gastric cancers raises hope that, through screening and treatment, many cancers can be prevented with treatment. The issue is more complex, however, and research looking into this is still in its infancy. One issue is the large number of asymptomatic infections. Roughly 30 percent of adults in the United States and 50 percent worldwide are infected with *H. pylori*. Whether treating this vast number of people who are infected but have no symptoms of gastritis or peptic ulcer disease could lower the risk of cancer is unknown and would be extremely costly. Currently, screening is done and treatment recommended primarily for those people diagnosed with gastritis or peptic ulcer disease.

Information on primary prevention of infection is also lacking although a few commonsense modalities, though speculative, may help. It is felt that *H. pylori* is acquired through person-to-person contact and via ingesting contaminated water and food. Some studies of well water have shown that *H. pylori* may be a contaminant around 65 percent of the time. Careful hand washing and filtering well water may decrease exposure. Babies who are breastfed are less likely to become infected as well. Historically, the decline in gastric cancer in the United States could shadow improvements in the water supply, but this is only speculation. Adequate intake of fruits and vegetables likely plays a role as well, and the lower the level of vitamin C in a person's blood, the more likely the person will become infected with *H. pylori*.

Diagnosis and treatment of *H. pylori* in the setting of peptic ulcer disease does make a difference. Traditional "ulcer" medications can alleviate the symptoms of ulcers due to *H. pylori*, but they frequently reoccur unless the infection is treated with a combination regimen of antibiotics. *H. pylori* can be diagnosed with a blood test, a breath test (which is more accurate), or tests done during endoscopy to look for ulcers. Eight treatment regimens are now approved by the FDA if an infection is diagnosed, which can resolve the majority of infections.

The question remains whether eradication of infection can lower the risk of cancer in addition to decreasing the recurrence of ulcers. In a study in China, it was found that treatment of *H. pylori* carriers without precancerous lesions lowered their risk of gastric cancer, providing hope that this could be the case (Wong, 2004). A vaccine has been developed that is effective in preventing infection in experimental animals, but studies on humans are a long way off.

Prostate Cancer: An Infectious Disease?

Epidemiological studies in the past have shown that men with a history of prostate infections are at increased risk of being diagnosed with prostate cancer. Prostate infections are generally considered bacterial and are treated with antibiotics. Men should seek prompt treatment if they are experiencing symptoms of a prostate infection, such as pain when urinating, and should undergo appropriate treatment.

A recent study at the Cleveland Clinic identified a retrovirus in men genetically predisposed to prostate cancer (Klein, 2006). It is unknown if this virus causes prostate symptoms or has any association with the prostate infections mentioned above. Further, it isn't known how it is contracted, since this is a very recent discovery. If this virus is found to have a causative role in some cases of prostate cancer, which is merely speculation at this time, it does provide hope that primary prevention through avoidance of infection and immunization may be on the horizon.

Practical Points

- ❑ Hepatitis B vaccination is recommended for all children, adolescents, and high-risk adults. Since many infections occur in individuals without risk factors, immunization of all adults may be considered.
- ❑ If you had a blood transfusion (or have a sexual partner who did) prior to 1989, have ever used illegal injectable drugs, or have had abnormal liver tests, request a test for hepatitis C.
- ❑ Practice safe sex.
- ❑ Adolescent girls and sexually active women not in monogamous relationships should consider getting the HPV vaccine.
- ❑ If you develop infectious mononucleosis, take extra care with your health and diet.
- ❑ If you travel overseas, research the areas you will be traveling to for information about infections endemic to the region, and take appropriate precautions.
- ❑ If you have gastritis or peptic ulcer disease, see a physician and request a test for *H. pylori*.

Resources and Further Online Information

Center for Disease Control and Prevention. Traveler's Health

www.cdc.gov/travel/

The CDC offers this site, which provides information on infections that are prevalent based on your destinations. It also provides up-to-date information on outbreaks of infectious diseases around the world.

Hepatitis B Foundation

www.hepb.org/

This comprehensive Web site contains information on the diagnosis, prevention, and treatment of hepatitis B.

Medline Plus. Hepatitis C

www.nlm.nih.gov/medlineplus/hepatitisc.html

The National Library of Medicine and the National Institute of Medicine provide this excellent site, with information ranging from a general overview of hepatitis C to nutrition and alternative therapy for those who are infected with the virus.

Centers for Disease Control and Prevention. HIV/AIDS. Fact Sheets

www.cdc.gov/hiv/resources/factsheets/index.htm

This CDC site contains extensive information about HIV/AIDS, with a focus on prevention.

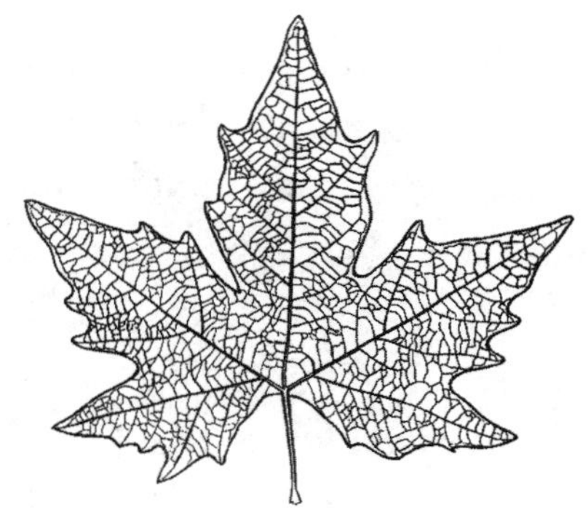

Chapter Six

Lifestyle and Cancer Prevention

"The best six doctors anywhere
And no one can deny it
Are sunshine, water, rest and air
Exercise and diet.
These six will gladly you attend
If only you are willing
Your mind they'll ease
Your will they'll mend
And charge you not a shilling."

—Nursery rhyme quoted by Wayne Fields, *What the River Knows*, 1990

Like a rose thorn in the thumb that eludes a tweezers, reasons why the life expectancy in a dozen major European countries is higher than that in the U.S. have been difficult to discern. Life expectancy in Norway, France, Austria, Finland, Switzerland, Italy, Spain, and Germany, to name a few, is higher than in the United States even though their rate of smoking is higher. There are more smokers in Japan and Australia as well, and residents there live longer than those that reside in the U.S. Greece has the highest rate of smoking in the world, yet the Greeks live longer than the average American!

The subject of tobacco use is **not** under debate. It has been shown beyond a shadow of a doubt that smoking causes cancer and kills prematurely. Our question is, if Greeks, say, did not smoke, would the gap between their life expectancy and ours be greater still? Probably, given what we know about smoking, but why? What are they doing that we in the United States are not?

Could it have anything to do with the average American walking a fraction of the distance the typical European does daily? Could it have anything to do with the casual observation that while walking through the Amsterdam airport to reach connecting flights, the authors couldn't really find an overweight person, while in the United States, we simply need to open our eyes to see several overweight people instantly? Could it have anything to do with the typical European vacationing from the stress of work for a few months each year instead of the few weeks a typical U.S. citizen is granted?

We begin our discussion of lifestyle factors with a discussion of tobacco, since it is the number one cause of cancer in the United States, but as we see clearly through life-expectancy statistics, cancer prevention goes far beyond smoking cessation. Information on the hazards of smoking has been extensively publicized and many excellent resources are available to help those dedicated to quitting, so our emphasis in this chapter will be on lifestyle factors in addition to smoking that predispose a person to develop or help a person to prevent cancer.

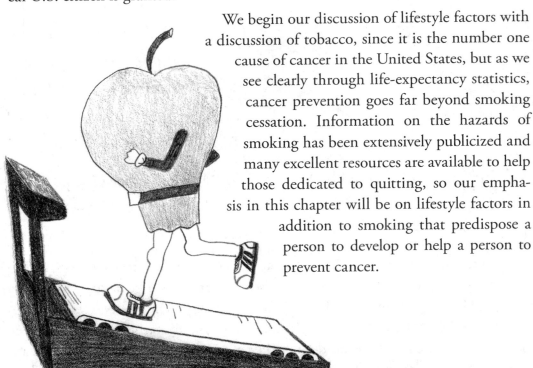

SMOKING/TOBACCO

"One thousand Americans stop smoking everyday – by dying."

—Author unknown

"Cancer cures smoking."

—Author unknown

Tobacco use is the number one cause of preventable cancer in the United States, accounting for 30 percent of all cancers. Eighty-seven percent of lung cancers are attributed to smoking alone. Tobacco use can also cause cancer of the kidney, bladder, pancreas, and stomach, as well as acute myelogenous leukemia. Smoking during pregnancy may increase the risk of childhood leukemia in children genetically predisposed, and exposure to the fifty-plus carcinogens that are released into the air with lighting a cigarette leaves those exposed non-smokers two to three times more likely to develop lung cancer than those not exposed. Though the rate of smoking has declined through widespread recognition of the risks, an amazing number of our teens still take up the habit. More than 6.4 million children living in the Unites States today are estimated to die prematurely in the future because of the decision to begin smoking as adolescents today.

If you smoke and need assistance, many resources are available to help you kick the habit. In addition to brochures, classes, and support groups, other resources are available. Nicotine replacement therapy through the use of a patch, gum, nasal spray, or inhaler is available, with many products sold over the counter now without a prescription. The medication Zyban® has been approved to decrease cravings.

The Center for Disease Control (CDC) has developed an excellent motivational tool that depicts how rapidly quitting smoking begins to make a difference in one's health. Table 6-1 is a poster published by the CDC as part of its Tobacco Information and Prevention Source (TIPS), and can be accessed online at www.cdc.gov/tobacco/sgr/sgr_2004/posters/20mins.htm. This can be a positive reminder to those trying to quit smoking as they struggle through the first few months. Several numbers and Internet resources are listed at the end of this chapter that provide many suggestions for facilitating the quitting process.

Table 6-1. Within 20 Minutes of Quitting

WITHIN 20 MINUTES AFTER YOU SMOKE THAT LAST CIGARETTE, YOUR BODY BEGINS A SERIES OF CHANGES THAT CONTINUE FOR YEARS.

20 Minutes After Quitting
Your heart rate drops.

12 Hours After Quitting
Carbon monoxide level in your blood drops to normal.

2 Weeks to 3 Months After Quitting
Your heart attack risk begins to drop.
Your lung function begins to improve.

1 to 9 Months After Quitting
Your coughing and shortness of breath decrease.

1 Year After Quitting
Your added risk of coronary heart disease is half that of a smoker's.

5 Years After Quitting
Your stroke risk is reduced to that of a nonsmoker's 5-15 years after quitting.

10 Years After Quitting
Your lung cancer death rate is about half that of a smoker's.
Your risk of cancers of the mouth, throat, esophagus, bladder, kidney, and pancreas decreases.

15 Years After Quitting
Your risk of coronary heart disease is back to that of a nonsmoker's.

Source: Centers for Disease Control and Prevention. CDC Tobacco Information and Prevention Source (TIPS) Available at www.cdc.gov/tobacco/how2quit.htm.

Who in the world is doing all the smoking anyway? As Figure 6-1 shows, the U.S. has one of the lowest percentages of citizens who smoke daily, no doubt due to the anti-smoking campaigns in place since the mid 1970s. And countries like Greece and Japan, without similar campaigns, have several of the highest. Even in the U.S. what can non-smokers do to make a difference? If your favorite establishments allow smoking, make your voice heard. The more often owners hear complaints, the more likely they will be to address the issue. To protect yourself, avoid places where you will be exposed to secondhand smoke. Do not allow your family and friends to smoke around you and continue to remind them to quit smoking. The more often the negative aspects of smoking enter their conscious thought, the more likely they will be to quit. If you hesitate because you are afraid of offending them, think of it as reminding them to move if they are standing in oncoming traffic looking the wrong way!

CIGARS

Cigars have gained popularity recently since the risk of lung cancer is somewhat lower when smoking cigars than with cigarettes, yet cigar smokers continue to have higher rates of lung cancer than nonsmokers do, and are four to ten times more likely to die from cancers of the esophagus, mouth, and larynx than nonsmokers are. In addition, second-hand smoke from cigars is just as dangerous to nonsmokers as that from cigarettes.

CHEWING TOBACCO

People that use smokeless tobacco are at an increased risk for cancers of the mouth, lip, tongue, gums, and cheeks. Our children may not see chewing in the same light as smoking, especially when they see their idealized athletes spitting on the baseball fields. Perhaps we should point out to them that Babe Ruth died at the young age of fifty-two from oropharyngeal cancer (cancer in the back of the throat) most likely due to chewing tobacco. If you or a loved one needs help quitting, information about the NSTEP program, a very thorough resource, is listed at the end of this chapter.

MARIJUANA

In addition to its being illegal, marijuana poses a cancer risk especially to those that use this drug during pregnancy. Marijuana has been shown to cause cancer in animals, and there is a significant association between children born to mothers who used marijuana and the risk of rhabdomyosarcoma (a soft tissue cancer) and one type of leukemia in those children (Grufferman, 1993).

Figure 6-1 Regular Smoking by Country

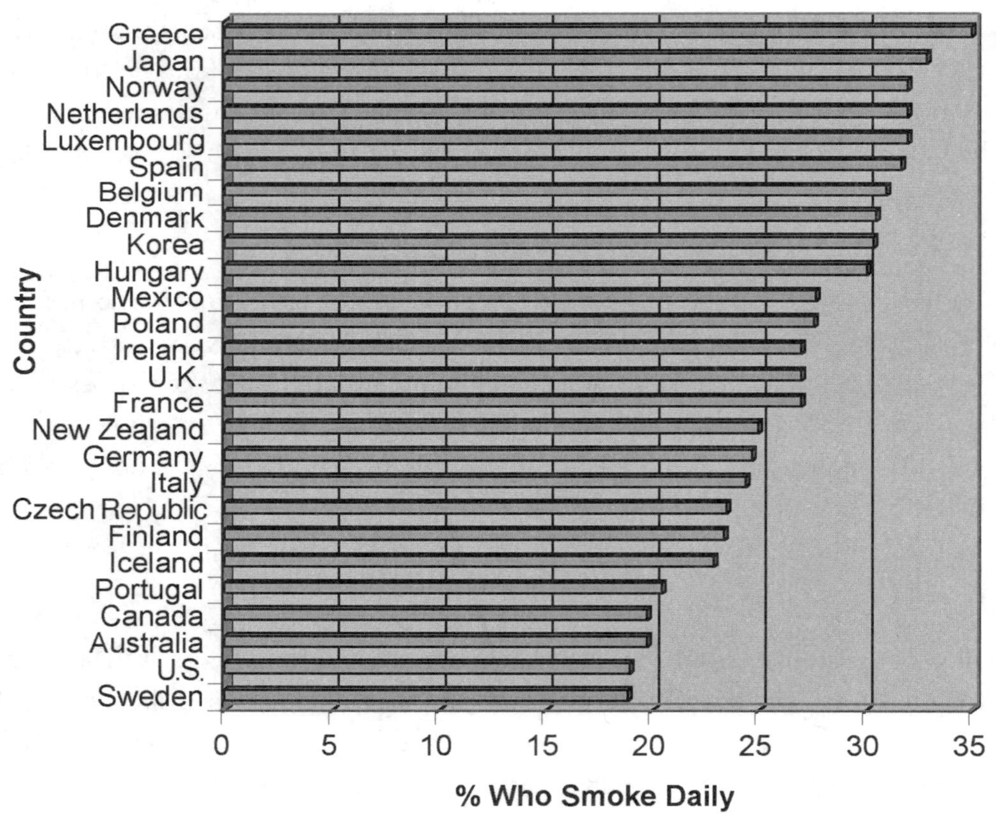

Source: OECD Health Data 2003.

OBESITY

"Thou seest I have more flesh than another man, and therefore more frailty."
—William Shakespeare

After smoking, obesity is the second leading preventable cause of cancer in the United States. If trends continue, we predict that obesity will soon sprint ahead to take over first place in the race for the hangman trophy. As smoking declines, obesity perseveres, and in fact has relentlessly increased over the past few decades. The percent of obese adult Americans has doubled in the last twenty-five years, and is now over 30 percent of the population (see Figure 6-2). Comparing data from 1999-2000 with that from 2003-2004 alone, the prevalence of overweight and obese male children rose from 14.0 to 18.2 percent, and that of female children from 13.8 to 16.0 percent. Currently 78.2 percent of men aged forty to fifty-nine in the United States are overweight or obese (Ogden, 2006). If child psychologists are correct in their thinking that children learn more from their parents' actions than their words, the forecast for obesity rates has gone from partly cloudy to severe storm warnings. When will we be prepared enough to predict the devastation and sound the sirens?

Looking at the statistics regarding obesity imparts a sense of futility and resignation. According to a CDC study in 2005 (Flegal, 2005), the number of excess deaths in the U.S. associated with obesity "is equivalent to a jetliner full of 300 people crashing every day" (National Alliance for Nutrition and Activity, 2006, 6). The future of obesity does not have to inspire the same sense of foreboding as might threats of global warming, however we **do** have some control over the weight of our county.

Perhaps we need to consider thoughtfully what empowered our nation to rise up and launch an attack on smoking, an effective ambush that has left tobacco retreating. When will we see anti-obesity campaigns on commercials during our prime time shows? When will we see the fast food industry follow the Phillip Morris example and contribute to prevention while they make their money from our ignorance? When will those of us in the U.S who take pride in living in the country that has by far the highest health care expenditure per person in the world

Figure 6-2 Obesity by Country

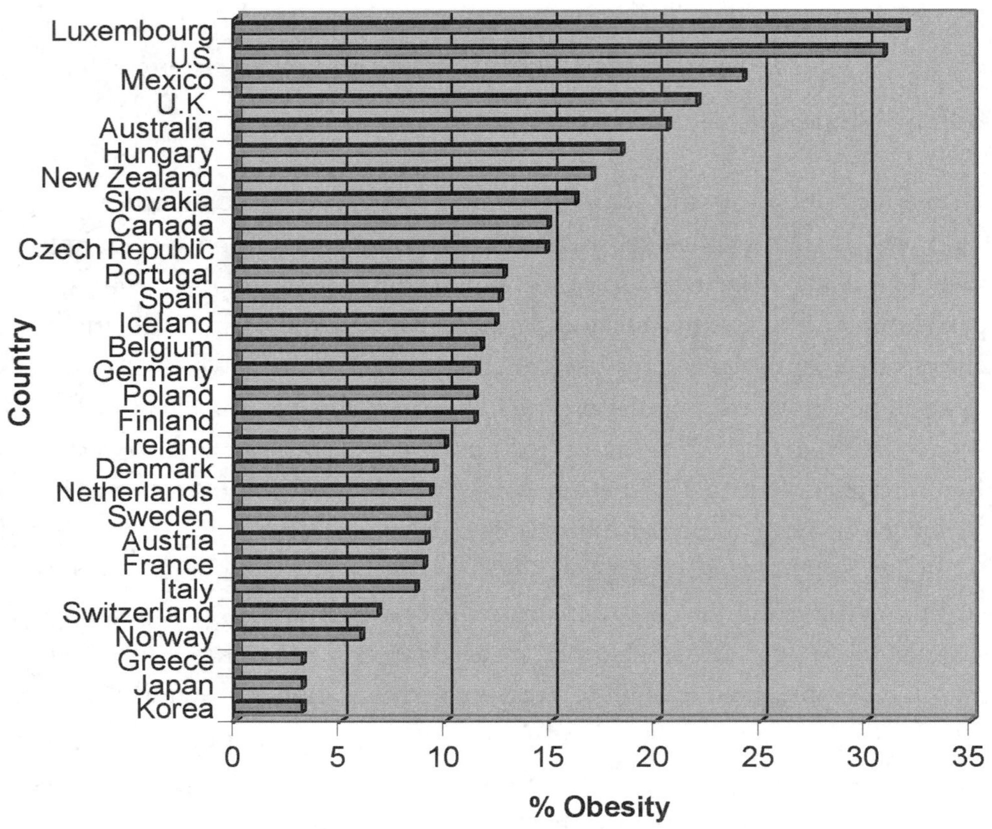

Source: OECD Health Data 2003.

become enraged that our life expectancy does not even make the top forty, and actively seek out the reasons and cures? When will we become saddened enough that a decline in our life expectancy has been predicted, and due to obesity, we are now expected to live **longer** than our children (Olshansky, 2005)?

We subsidize the production of corn in our country, but what products are produced from corn? Most corn is used to produce low quality foods with sugar as the number one ingredient. Perhaps we should instead be subsidizing the production of other vegetables and fruits.

We hear reports about the cost of smoking and the billions of healthcare dollars spent each year for smoking-related illnesses. If our predictions are correct, obesity may be more costly than smoking in the near future. Part of the argument against smoking includes the risk to "secondhand smokers." While being obese or overweight does not double or triple the risk of developing cancer for non-obese loved ones as their exposure to cigarette smoke does, we would argue that it does affect more than the obese individual.

Those of us who are not overweight have a job to do as well. We need to offer encouragement when we see someone that is overweight exercising and eating a healthy diet, just as we praise our friends that have succeeded in quitting smoking.

Why are we growing wider?

For all medical disorders, we need to understand causes to find effective treatments. Vaccines cannot be developed until we know the microbe we are fighting. High blood pressure cannot be treated until we understand the hormonal and chemical processes in the body that contribute to the diagnosis. An imminent heart attack cannot be prevented until we are aware of the artery that is clogged, place a stent, and also address the multiple factors that worked together to create the obstruction in the first place. In order to offer an effective treatment for obesity, we likewise need to understand the underlying causes and examine contributing factors before we can develop an informed treatment plan.

While many underlying causes and contributing factors jump to mind based on an international perspective, we would venture to guess that the number one cause of our growing waistlines in the U.S. is portion distortion. Research has shown that over the last few decades the average portion of food served at most restaurants has increased dramatically. This began to happen long before we were "super-sized." We are served greater portions at restaurants and, following their example, begin to serve more at home. If anyone should question this theory, we would ask him or her to visit a few restaurants in European countries, where obesity is less common. The average portions served, and even the size of soft drinks and french fries at fast food restaurants, in Europe is smaller.

In the United States, women are consuming 335 more calories per day and men 168 calories more than they did thirty years ago (Wright, 2004). To understand the impact of this, an extra 100 calories per day translates into ten pounds per year. To work off an extra 100 calories per day would require walking twenty-five minutes a day. To simply maintain her weight (not lose), a typical American woman would have to walk seventy-five minutes a day **more** than she did thirty years ago!

Fast food is also a villain, but is not the only cause of our struggle with obesity. Fast food is available in countries where obesity is much less common, though the portions are smaller, as noted previously. Fast food is described at greater length in the discussion of nutrition in Chapter Eight, but note that those individuals who eat two or more times a week at fast food establishments are 50 percent more likely to be overweight or obese than are individuals who don't (Pereira, 2005). Dining on fast food can have long-term ramifications as well. Young adults who eat frequently at fast food restaurants gain more weight and have a greater increase in insulin resistance in middle age than those who do not.

Peer pressure probably plays a significant role, although in a different form than we are accustomed to. Since the majority of our population is overweight or obese, it is often viewed as "acceptable" to carry those extra pounds. Perhaps a **lack** of peer pressure is the problem here. If someone is a part of the majority party that carries the vote, there is little incentive to change preferences. What if someone from this party transfers to another region, where they are now in the minority with little support and comradery? Won't this person feel pressure to change his or her ways? What if an overweight person from the United States should find themselves in Asia or Europe? Would there then be incentive and initiative to join the norm? In the United States, individuals can be overweight and remain in their comfort zone.

Lack of exercise is clearly a significant reason. Compared to much of the world, we are a sedentary society. Easy access to motorized transportation allows us to rest our legs while we head to the store or out to see friends. When we return home, we have television, computer games, and video games to help us relax further.

Statistics tell us being overweight or obese accounts for 20 percent of cancers in women and 14 percent of cancers in men, raising the risk of developing colon, postmenopausal breast, uterine, esophageal, and kidney cancers (Calle, 2003;

Bianchini, 2002). Some studies suggest that once an overweight individual develops cancer they have a higher risk of recurrence and poorer survival (McTiernan, 2005). Being overweight clearly raises the risk of having complications from surgery and other treatments, such as the development of clots in the legs and the slow healing of wounds.

How does being overweight affect cancer risk?

Excess weight plays a role in the development of cancer in several ways. Researchers have been evaluating the connection between sex steroids, such as estrogen, insulin growth factor, and insulin, and the possible connection with cancer. Elevated estrogen levels related to excess body mass are considered a reason for the increased incidence of breast cancer in postmenopausal obese women. Being overweight or obese is the cause of roughly 80 percent of diabetes, and diabetes is a risk factor for cancer (see our discussion about diabetes in Chapter Seven). Further, being overweight or obese also increases the risk of having gallstones, the primary risk factor for gallbladder cancer.

Weight management

A comprehensive discussion of weight management is beyond the scope of this book, but we offer a few suggestions. If your body mass index is over twenty-five (see Figure 6-3), we strongly recommend talking with your healthcare provider and working with him or her to design a program to help you reduce your weight. It is important to prepare and make a long-term commitment to not only losing those extra pounds, but also maintaining any weight loss you achieve over time. "Yo-yo" dieting (repeatedly losing and regaining weight) may have a lasting negative effect on the immune system (Shade, 2004).

Figure 6-3 Body Mass Index Chart

BMI	Height (in)																		
	58	**59**	**60**	**61**	**62**	**63**	**64**	**65**	**66**	**67**	**68**	**69**	**70**	**71**	**72**	**73**	**74**	**75**	**76**
Wgt. (lbs)	4'10"	4'11"	5'0"	5'1"	5'2"	5'3"	5'4"	5'5"	5'6"	5'7"	5'8"	5'9"	5'10"	5'11"	6'0"	6'1'	6'2"	6'3'	6'4'
100	21	20	20	19	18	18	17	17	16	16	15	15	14	14	14	13	13	13	12
105	22	21	21	20	19	19	18	18	17	16	16	16	15	15	14	14	14	13	13
110	23	22	22	21	20	20	19	18	18	17	17	16	16	15	15	15	14	14	13
115	24	23	23	22	21	20	20	19	19	18	18	17	17	16	16	15	15	14	14
120	25	24	23	23	22	21	21	20	19	19	18	18	17	17	16	16	15	15	15
125	26	25	24	24	23	22	22	21	20	20	19	18	18	17	17	17	16	16	15
130	27	26	25	25	24	23	22	22	21	20	20	19	19	18	18	17	17	16	16
135	28	27	26	26	25	24	23	23	22	21	21	20	19	19	18	18	17	17	16
140	29	28	27	27	26	25	24	23	23	22	21	21	20	20	19	19	18	18	17
145	30	29	28	27	27	26	25	24	23	23	22	21	21	20	20	19	19	18	18
150	31	30	29	28	27	27	26	25	24	24	23	22	22	21	20	20	19	19	18
155	32	31	30	29	28	28	27	26	25	24	24	23	22	22	21	20	20	19	19
160	34	32	31	30	29	28	28	27	26	25	24	24	23	22	22	21	21	20	20
165	35	33	32	31	30	29	28	28	27	26	25	24	24	23	22	22	21	21	20
170	36	34	33	32	31	30	29	28	27	27	26	25	24	24	23	22	22	21	21
175	37	35	34	33	32	31	30	29	28	27	27	26	25	24	24	23	23	22	21
180	38	36	35	34	33	32	31	30	29	28	27	27	26	25	24	24	23	23	22
185	39	37	36	35	34	33	32	31	30	29	28	27	27	26	25	24	24	23	23
190	40	38	37	36	35	34	33	32	31	30	29	28	27	27	26	25	24	24	23
195	41	39	38	37	36	35	34	33	32	31	30	29	28	27	27	26	25	24	24
200	42	40	39	38	37	36	34	33	32	31	30	30	29	28	27	26	26	25	24
205	43	41	40	39	38	36	35	34	33	32	31	30	29	29	28	27	26	26	25
210	44	43	41	40	38	37	36	35	34	33	32	31	30	29	29	28	27	26	26
215	45	44	42	41	39	38	37	36	35	34	33	32	31	30	29	28	28	27	26
220	46	45	43	42	40	39	38	37	36	35	34	33	32	31	30	29	28	28	27
225	47	46	44	43	41	40	39	38	36	35	34	33	32	31	31	30	29	28	27
230	48	47	45	44	42	41	40	38	37	36	35	34	33	32	31	30	30	29	28
235	49	48	46	44	43	42	40	39	38	37	36	35	34	33	32	31	30	29	29
240	50	49	47	45	44	43	41	40	39	38	37	36	35	34	33	32	31	30	29
245	51	50	48	46	45	43	42	41	40	38	37	36	35	34	33	32	32	31	30
250	52	51	49	47	46	44	43	42	40	39	38	37	36	35	34	33	32	31	30
255	53	52	50	48	47	45	44	43	41	40	39	38	37	36	35	34	33	32	31
260	54	53	51	49	48	46	45	43	42	41	40	38	37	36	35	34	33	33	32
265	56	54	52	50	49	47	46	44	43	42	40	39	38	37	36	35	34	33	32
270	57	55	53	51	49	48	46	45	44	42	41	40	39	38	37	36	35	34	33
275	58	56	54	52	50	49													

BMI	CATEGORY	WAIST LESS THAN OR EQUAL TO 40" (MEN) OR 35" (WOMEN)	WAIST GREATER THAN 40" (MEN) OR 35" (WOMEN)
18.5 or less	Underweight	N/A	N/A
18.5 - 24.9	Normal	N/A	N/A
25.0 - 29.9	Overweight	Increased Risk	High Risk
30.0 - 34.9	Obese	High Risk	Very High Risk
35.0 - 39.9	Obese	Very High Risk	Very High Risk
40 or greater	Extremely Obese	Extremely High Risk	Extremely High Risk

Practical tips on managing your weight:

- Be aware of unconscious eating. Do not eat while watching TV or reading.
- Do not skip breakfast.
- Use smaller plates.
- Keep a detailed journal of what you eat. Knowing you have to write it down may help you pass by a few high-calorie items.
- Eat high-fiber foods such as legumes and apples so you feel full.
- When you are full, stop eating. If you feel bad wasting food and remember the posters from elementary school of children starving in the world, make a note to put less on your plate next time. Instead, transfer your concern to your body, which can likewise suffer from overeating.
- Become active. Read our tips on exercise below. Turn off the computer and TV and go for a walk.
- Graze. Eat less more often to keep your metabolism in check and to avoid becoming ravenously hungry and not caring as much about the calories you ingest.
- Allow yourself to indulge in a few taboo foods on occasion. You will be much more likely to stick with a program if it is not too prohibitive.
- Eat slowly. If you find this hard, try eating with your non-dominant hand to slow you down.
- Bring your lunch to work.
- Stay busy to avoid eating out of boredom.
- Avoid all soft drinks, including diet varieties. Choose bottled water, iced tea, and, on occasion, 100-percent fruit juice or milk as an alternative.
- Choose healthy snacks rather than high-calorie snack foods and chips. Good choices include carrot and celery sticks, fresh vegetables, and low-fat dried fruits.

- Always eat and have a full stomach prior to grocery shopping.
- Serve food at home as restaurants do. Place food on plates without having serving dishes available to take "seconds."
- Sign up for a yoga class. Yoga helps limit weight gain in middle age.
- Keep a list of the reasons you want to achieve or maintain a healthy weight on the refrigerator.
- If you are overweight but do not have diabetes, familiarize yourself with the diabetic diet and try to follow it.

Tips on Eating Out:

- Ask for sauces, dressings, and mayo "on the side."
- Do not "supersize."
- Avoid fried foods; instead, choose foods that are baked, broiled, or roasted.
- Skip dessert or order fresh fruit.
- Eat a little something before you go out so you are not extremely hungry.
- Limit your intake of bread and chips while awaiting your meal.
- Order the smallest portion possible, such as the petite steak, or a quarter-pound burger instead of the third- or half-pound choices.
- When ordering soups choose broth-based rather than cream-based soups.
- Be aware of portions. Choose a child's portion if possible or split a meal with a friend.
- Limit selections that contain cheese.
- Do not order a portion greater than your caloric requirement allows. Many people order large dishes, planning to take some home for another meal. The problem, however, is that they often end up eating much more than they would otherwise. Studies repeatedly show that if we have more on our plate we will eat significantly more.

The end of this chapter lists resources such as Weight Watchers™ that can be helpful for those who struggle with obesity. Whether the resources you use are through a program like this, your healthcare provider, or on your own, make sure you are accountable to someone who can provide encouragement along the way.

EXERCISE/PHYSICAL ACTIVITY

"Physical fitness is not only one of the keys to a healthy body, it is the basis of dynamic and creative intellectual activity."

—John F. Kennedy

Figure 6-4 Obesity vs. Physical Activity by Country

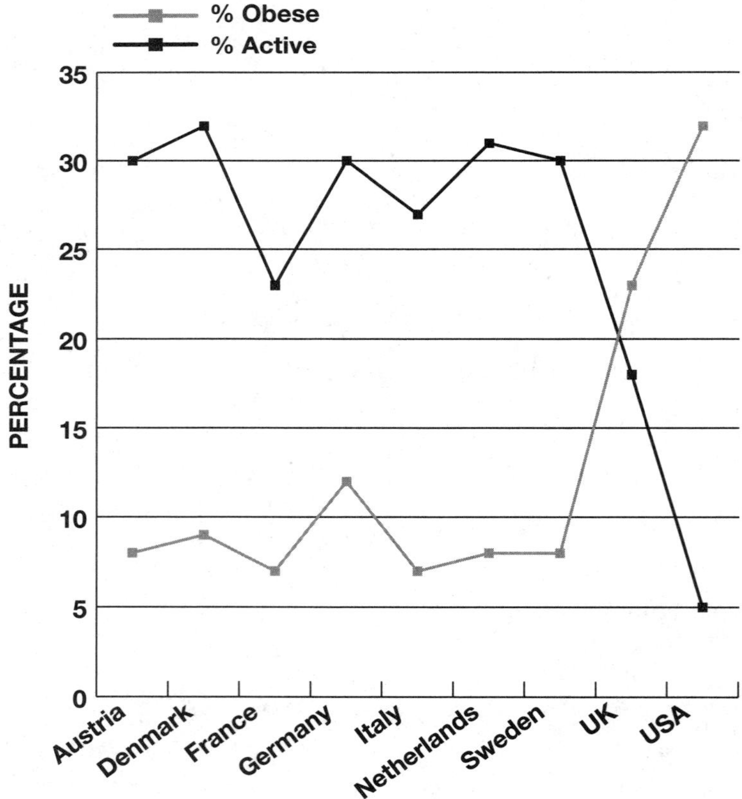

Source: Rutgers University. Available at http://policy.rutgers.edu/faculty/pucher.htm.

One solution for gaining control of our obesity epidemic and subsequent cancer risk in the U.S. is to improve our nation's fitness (see Figure 6-4). Of the countries listed in this figure, the U.S. has the lowest life expectancy. Many studies have demonstrated the benefit of exercise in reducing the risk of developing cancer, some showing significant benefit with even very modest increases in daily activity (Lee, 2003; Friedenreich, 2002). The American Cancer Society recommends thirty minutes of physical activity or more on five or more days per week for adults. Increasing this to forty-five minutes per day of moderate to vigorous activity on five or more days per week seems to enhance the decreases seen in breast and colon cancer. Physical activity to reduce cancer risk does not require a pricey health club membership and could actually save you money. Activities such as washing windows, raking, and vacuuming qualify. Here are a few ideas to increase your activity level:

- Purchase a pedometer and see how many steps you can take in a day. To improve your motivation and accountability, find a friend, coworker, or child to do the same and compare "mileage."
- Park as far as possible from your destination and walk (this will also free up the closest parking spaces for those who really need them).
- Help elderly neighbors rake their yards or weed their gardens.
- Avoid elevators and use the stairs.
- When you travel, make use of the hotel's fitness room.
- Go dancing.
- Sign up for an exercise class, yoga, or pilates, and commit to attending it. Find a partner to exercise with so you are accountable.
- Write in "exercise" on your daily calendar/to-do list.
- Travel to Europe and try to walk as the Europeans do.
- Think about your lifestyle as someone observing you would. Be honest. If you were another person evaluating your lifestyle and activity level, what suggestions would you make for change? Think about them.
- If you would like extra motivation, adults can earn Presidential Fitness Awards like the one children do in school! If you log at least thirty

minutes of exercise five days a week you can earn a Presidential Active Lifestyle Award. Information is available on the President's Challenge Web site accessible at www.presidentschallenge.org/pdf/active_lifestyle.pdf.

Physical Activity In Children

Physical activity in twelve to twenty-four-year-old females was shown to significantly reduce the risk of their developing breast cancer (Lagerros, 2004). This is frightening in an age when time for physical activity is being filled with time at the computer or watching cable TV. From observing the amount of time the average preteen and adolescent spends watching TV, text messaging their friends on their cell phones, and conversing on the phone, by email and by instant messaging, we contend that many children fall far below the daily recommended dose of exercise. In 1999, when fewer children had cell phones, and text messaging was still a toddler, a study found that children spent an average of 6 hours 32 minutes **daily** with various media combined (Roberts, 1999). The American Cancer Society recommends that children and adolescents engage in at least sixty minutes of moderate to vigorous activity five days per week. In this day when expensive health club memberships are so popular, we forget that children were much more physically fit before fitness clubs spanned the nation. In countries such as Sweden where health clubs are few and far between, children are much fitter and less overweight than are those in the U.S. (Vincent, 2003). Instead of running outside chasing butterflies, jumping in puddles, having casual games of baseball in the neighborhood, and climbing trees, many of our children are watching other children play on TV.

The number one priority in improving the fitness of our children is to improve our own physical fitness. Children learn from our actions, not just from our words. If we exercise regularly and maintain a healthy weight, they will learn to do likewise. If we tell them to be active and not overeat, but have a sedentary lifestyle and gain unhealthy pounds ourselves, they will most likely turn out the same.

A FEW IDEAS FOR INCREASING ACTIVITY IN CHILDREN

- Make exercise FUN, not a chore.
- Make sure that children see that exercise is a priority in your life.
- Walk together; explore together.
- "Tolerate" your children's music and dance with them.
- Pick out activities that require walking, whether it is a hike in the mountains, by a lake, or walking around a science museum.
- Park the car in a distant parking space when shopping or going to activities with your children. You can use this as an opportunity to reinforce the importance of exercise, as well as to share with them a generous spirit, letting them know you are "saving" those nearby parking spaces for someone who is elderly or has difficulty walking as far.
- Be involved when your children participate in the Presidential Physical Fitness Award at school. Ask them their numbers (like how many sit-ups they could do) so they know you are interested. Do not push them beyond reason, but let them know you value exercise.
- Encourage sports activities that they are interested in, but within reason. Children need time to be children and simply play.
- Purchase birthday and Christmas presents designed to promote exercise. A few ideas include: bicycles, balls, jump ropes, badminton or volleyball nets and equipment, a ping pong table, tennis racquets, hula hoops, a baton, skates, a Frisbee, kites, juggling balls, a basketball hoop, chalk to draw lines to play hopscotch, running shoes, goggles for swimming, or a dog they will be required to walk daily.
- Limit TV, video games, and computer time and stick with it.
- Play tennis as a family. To keep this fun and non-competitive with young children, "score" by counting the number of times the ball can go over the net in a row.

- Plan active family vacations; go to a national park and hike; plan a canoe trip.

Is your child's school a "fit" school? Obesity in children has doubled in the last few decades, and playing active outdoor activities is frequently replaced by staring at a screen of some form at home. So what activity is your child getting at school? In many cases physical education taught in school has declined and been replaced by more sedentary activities, while school lunches have become more processed and caloric. Check to see if your state provides any incentive to schools to emphasize fitness and, if not, suggest that they begin one. In Minnesota, the governor has created a "Governor's Fitness Challenge." Schools in the state can apply to become a "Governor's Fit School" if they meet standards based on opportunities for physical activity during the day as well as certain meal standards.

Stress and Cancer

"Worry and stress affects the circulation, the heart, the glands, the whole nervous system, and profoundly affects heart action."

—Charles W. Mayo

Until fairly recently, depression, anxiety, and emotional distress due to stressful life events were considered purely psychological phenomena by Western medicine. Events such as the loss of a loved one, divorce, social isolation, and loneliness were recognized for their emotional impact, but little was known about how these tragedies affected the body physiologically. Research is now bringing to light information about how the mind affects the endocrine (glands that secrete hormones) and immune systems, and thereby its potential role in inducing or preventing cancer or other diseases.

Understanding what studies say about the relation between our emotions and health requires talking about our nervous system's design. The nervous system is divided into two parts, the central nervous system (consisting of the brain and spinal cord) and the peripheral nervous system, which carries information from the rest of the body to and from the central nervous system. The peripheral nervous system is in turn divided into the somatic nervous system responsible for **conscious** responses, such as those of our five senses and movement, and the autonomic nervous system, which is again divided into the sympathetic and parasympathetic systems. It is at the level of the autonomic nervous system, which is responsible for **unconscious** responses such as heartbeat and the secretion of hormones by endocrine glands, that stress can affect our bodily functions.

Historically, our sympathetic nervous system responded to physical stressors (for example, being attacked by a lion) by releasing stress hormones, increasing heart rate, respiratory rate and blood pressure; increasing blood sugar; increasing skeletal muscle contraction and excitation (to help us run from the lion); and increasing blood clotting factors (in case the lion bites us). In modern society, most stressors are psychological or interpersonal in nature. What used to help save our lives may now cost us our lives. For example, the increase in platelet aggregation (clotting) to help stop our bleeding from a lion bite now makes a heart attack more likely.

Daily stress results in chronic over-arousal of the sympathetic nervous system, which has been linked to immune suppression as well as dysfunction of the endocrine system. Stressful life events such as job changes and relationship breakups have been linked to a decrease in natural killer cells, a type of white blood cell in the immune system that finds and destroys tumor cells. Stress has also been linked to alterations in DNA repair and cell death, which have been shown to predispose to cancer. Clinically, stress has been correlated with developing cancer as well, and a study in Sweden found stress to be associated with a two-fold increase in the incidence of breast cancer in women, though these findings have not been replicated in other studies (Helgesson, 2003). Isolation and loneliness are risk factors for all types of disease, and a sense of belonging to a community can have a tremendous impact on both psychological and physical health.

Knowing that our emotional state can play a role in cancer predisposition or prevention, how can we practice primary prevention? Interacting with a supportive network of friends, meditating, praying, relaxing, and doing yoga, Qi Gong, and other such activities can help to break this cycle of sympathetic nervous system over-arousal, and thereby improve the effectiveness of the immune system in combating both infection and the development of cancers. These activities can calm the mind, toning down the "fight or flight" activity of the sympathetic nervous system and enhancing the "relaxation response" of the parasympathetic nervous system. This relaxation response slows the heart and respiratory rates, lowers blood pressure, causes the body to become less responsive to adrenaline, decreases oxygen consumption, and decreases blood sugar levels.

Yoga has been shown to drop baseline blood sugar levels as well as increase the effectiveness of insulin. Yoga also promotes the drainage of lymph, a fluid composed of infection-fighting white blood cells and waste products of cellular activity. The relaxation response derived from yoga can be as effective in altering physiological factors as B-blockers, a type of blood pressure medication that lowers blood pressure and heart rate. Research suggests that only ten to twenty minutes of these mind-centering and calming activities once or twice a day can increase the body's stress threshold for a full twenty-four hours.

Many experts in complimentary and alternative medicine, as well as experts at large cancer centers, believe that meditation may contribute to the prevention and treatment of cancers. One large study looking at utilization of medical care showed a 50 percent reduction in hospital admissions of patients with benign and malignant tumors who were involved in a transcendental meditation program (Orme-Johnson, 1987). Research has also found that mindfulness meditation was associated with increased levels of melatonin, a hormone secreted by the pineal gland in the brain (discussed in our section on sleep) that lowers estrogen levels and hence may lower the risk of developing breast cancer (Massion, 1995).

Attending religious services may play a role in cancer prevention. Several studies have shown a lower mortality rate among those who attend religious services, although cancer as a cause of death was not separated out in these studies (Oman, 2002; Oman, 1998; Strawbridge, 1997; Hummer, 1999). Attending religious services was also found to improve immune function in patients with advanced breast cancer, and in healthy older adults (Sephton, 2001; Koenig, 1997). While it could be argued that individuals who attend religious services have other lifestyle factors that influence their life expectancy, these studies deserve consideration in a cancer prevention lifestyle.

Praying may be considered a health practice in addition to a religious practice. A study published in the *British Medical Journal* found that both reciting a prayer (such as the rosary) and a yoga mantra resulted in physiological changes that are associated with favorable effects on cardiovascular and respiratory function (Bernardi, 2001). For more information on cancer and prayer, you can visit www.cancerprayerday.org.

Stress clearly has an effect on physiological processes that take place in the body, though its role in cancer is less clear. Fortunately, we can take the existing research findings and our own intuition that excessive chronic stress is not healthy, and strive for a lifestyle that does not contain unnecessary stress, and in which we deal with the inevitable stressors that we all face in more helpful ways.

Ways of Dealing with Stress

- Play music that relaxes you, brings back pleasant memories, or makes you happy.
- Set limits; learn how to say no.
- Choose your battles (this was the best advice that a neighbor gave one of the authors about raising four children).
- Cultivate friendships; choose positive friends that manage stress well in their own lives.
- Keep a journal or talk to a good friend to purge negative thoughts. A caution about journal writing: the purpose is to purge your thoughts, not perseverate on them!
- Turn off the news.
- Try yoga.
- Attend an inspiring religious service.
- Try to arrive everywhere you go ten minutes early.

- Set priorities.
- Keep active "to do" lists. List one should contain important items. List two can outline important but not time-critical items. List three can identify optional items. Throw away list three.
- Learn how to delegate.
- Find a quiet, peaceful place; listen to your breath and calm your mind.
- Declutter your life. If there is something you know you should toss but feel sentimental about, take a picture of it before pitching it.
- Get enough sleep.
- Try visualization. When in a stressful situation, picture yourself in your ideal situation beyond the current crisis.
- Read an uplifting book.
- Take a vacation.
- Write down ten things that are wonderful in your life, allowing nothing negative. Even in the worst situations, you can usually find at least ten things. Flush toilets, toilet paper, and clean water can head the list.

Take one hour in the next week, preferably with a good friend who knows you well, and list as many stressors in your life as you can. Pick one thing on the list you have the ability to change and brainstorm ways to modify it that you can implement immediately. Pick one thing on the list you cannot change and begin to accept it and let it go. Learn to laugh. Take time to play. Most importantly, develop a passion. A leading psychologist who has researched extensively the link between cancer and stress claims that the best stress reducer is having a satisfying life (LeShan, 1974). Whether it is climbing mountains, running a marathon, reading poetry, or playing an instrument quietly at home, find an activity that brings spice to your life.

ANGER

"Anyone can become angry, that is easy; but to be angry with the right person, and to the right degree, and at the right time, and for the right purpose, and in the right way, this is not within everybody's power, that is not easy."

—Aristotle

Repressing anger can damage the immune system and subsequently lead to cancer. Remember that anger is not necessarily bad and that good people get angry. Anger is a symptom indicating that in some way you are being harmed or your needs are not being met. Address it.

DEPRESSION

"A cheerful heart is good medicine, but a crushed spirit dries up the bones."

—Proverbs 17:22 (NIV)

Studies designed to determine whether or not clinical depression predisposes a person to develop cancer have yielded conflicting results. Some studies have demonstrated increased risk of developing several cancers in patients with histories of clinical depression, while other studies have failed to show any correlation. As noted previously, the purpose of this book is not to confirm or dispel studies, but only to provide the reader with information regarding substances and situations that may predispose a person to being diagnosed with cancer. Regardless of whether or not depression does cause cancer, those who suffer should seek treatment. Untreated depression can steal joy and life from people, not unlike cancer.

ALCOHOL

"Health – what my friends are drinking to before they fall down."
—Phyllis Diller

The use of alcohol has been associated with the development of several cancers, including those of the mouth, esophagus, liver, breast, colon, and rectum. Alcohol use during pregnancy has been linked with an increase in developing breast cancer in female offspring as well (Hilakivi-Clarke, 2004). The combination of drinking excess alcohol in conjunction with smoking is particularly dangerous. Overall, it is felt that alcohol causes around three percent of cancers in the United States.

Consuming alcohol can be a cancer risk in several ways. Chronic inflammation of the liver from alcohol abuse and subsequent alcoholic hepatitis and cirrhosis can set the stage for the development of cancer, just as chronic damage to the mouth and esophagus from alcohol (especially in combination with smoking) raises the risk of mutations as the body attempts to repair the damage. Chronic alcohol abuse predisposes the drinker to vitamin deficiencies, as calories obtained from food are replaced by those derived from alcohol. Declining levels of vitamin A, the B vitamins including folic acid, and vitamin E may be involved. Alcoholics are susceptible to infections that their non-alcoholic counterparts resist, and this immune suppression may allow cancer cells to grow without a fight. There is also mounting evidence that alcohol causes direct damage to DNA as well. Acetaldehyde, a suspected carcinogen formed as the body metabolizes alcohol, may react with natural compounds the body produces for cell growth, triggering a reaction that damages DNA. Alcohol can work together with other factors to raise the risk of cancer as well. Hepatitis B, hepatitis C, and hemochromatosis all increase the risk of having liver cancer, and some studies have shown this risk to be accentuated by consuming alcohol.

There are many studies touting the benefits of drinking red wine because of its component, resveratrol. While the authors recognize these studies, we are also hesitant to recommend this wholeheartedly because of the dangers that drinking in excess presents. If you feel comfortable that you are able to limit your intake to that compatible with cancer prevention, a glass of red wine may be of benefit. If not, the resveratrol can also be found in red grapes, grape juice, peanuts, blueberries, and cranberries, and it may be wise to skip the wine.

It is currently recommended that men consume no more than two alcoholic beverages per day and women no more than one. One drink is classified as twelve ounces of beer, five ounces of wine, or one and a half ounces of eighty-proof spirits (hard liquor). For those who choose to drink, an adequate intake of folic acid is important and appears to lower the risk of developing breast cancer in women who are moderate drinkers. Many people who consume too much alcohol, as with those who smoke, need assistance to quit. The Alcoholics Anonymous Web site listed in the resources at the end of this chapter provides information on alcohol abuse and can help you find resources available in your area.

Sleep Habits

"A good laugh and a long sleep are the best cures in the doctor's book."
—Irish Proverb

From optimal duration of sleep to turning out the lights, we are beginning to understand how circadian rhythms and hormones produced at night affect our health. The Cancer Prevention II Study of the American Cancer Society demonstrated an increased mortality for people who sleep more than eight hours or less than four hours per night, with an ideal sleep duration of seven hours (Kripke, 2002). Other studies have shown that people who sleep less than six or more than nine hours per night are more likely to develop diabetes, a risk factor for developing cancer (Gottlieb, 2005). A Finnish study revealed that duration of sleep was inversely proportional to the risk of developing breast cancer in women (Verkasalo, 2005), and was documented as well in the widely publicized nurses' health study (Schernhammer, 2006).

Why should sleep affect our risk of cancer?

Circadian rhythms, the twenty-four-hour patterns of our bodies' biological clock, probably play a role. Circadian rhythms influence many functions in our bodies from hormone production to body temperature to heart rate. Repeated studies have shown that heart attacks are more frequent in the morning and asthma attacks more frequent at night due to these rhythms. Regular circadian rhythms play a role in the regulation of the immune system in several ways as well. Female flight attendants have an increased rate of breast cancer possibly due to disruption of circadian rhythms (although other factors such as electromagnetic radiation could play a role) (Rynolds, 2002; Tokumaru, 2006).

Melatonin, a hormone produced by the pineal gland in the brain during darkness, most likely plays a significant role in these findings as well. Melatonin is known to decrease the production of estrogen, possibly explaining why a longer duration of sleep guards against breast cancer. Production of melatonin is maximal in total darkness. In one study, completely blind women had a 36 percent decreased risk of developing breast cancer (Kliekene, 2001). This rose to a 70 percent reduction in a later study. Women who work night shifts have a higher incidence of breast cancer (Schernhammer, 2001; Schernhammer, 2006). It is felt that this increase is due to the suppression of melatonin production by exposure to light at night. Recently night-shift work has been correlated with an increase in colon cancer in women as well (Schernhammer, 2006). Some studies have found that melatonin may improve survival among people with existing cancer (Mills, 2005). However, studies looking at the association between melatonin and breast cancer have been inconsistent, some showing an effect (Schernhammer, 2005), and others finding no evidence that the level of melatonin is associated with the risk of developing breast cancer. Carefully planned studies need to be completed to confirm the effectiveness and safety of melatonin in cancer treatment as well as to clarify its role in primary prevention. Yet, we should not wait years for the results of further studies to make adequate sleep in darkness a priority. This is the beauty of primary prevention: we do not have to wait for all of the answers before making lifestyle changes that we often know intuitively are healthy!

So what should you do if you are an insomniac? The use of prescription sleeping pills in these studies was associated with significantly increased mortality. If you suffer from sleep problems, it is crucial to discuss this with your physician.

Disorders such as sleep apnea are under-diagnosed and confer substantial risk if untreated. Sleep clinics are popping up around the country and can help to diagnose sleep apnea as well as disorders such as circadian rhythm disturbances. The subjective complaint of "insomnia" did not increase mortality, so do not lose more sleep worrying if this is the case! If you suffer from insomnia or poor sleep habits, we offer a few suggestions:

- Try to go to bed and get up at the same time every day regardless of whether it is a work day or the weekend.
- Quiet your mind a few hours before bedtime. Do not start new projects.
- Address serious issues earlier in the day. Do not "let the sun go down on your anger."
- Get exercise during the day.
- Avoid caffeine, alcohol, and tobacco. Alcohol may appear to help people fall asleep but they do not sleep as deeply.
- If you read at bedtime, make it light reading.
- Use the bedroom only for sleep and sex.
- TURN OFF THE LIGHTS.
- Avoid night lights; any light suppresses melatonin secretion.

A Healthy Sex Life

"Sex relieves tension – love causes it."

—Woody Allen

Using the bedroom for more than sleep can play a role in cancer prevention. Making a U-turn from the last chapter where we discussed the perils of unsafe sex and its role in cancer, we now discuss how a healthy sex life in a monogamous relationship may protect you from the frightening c-word. Conceptually it makes sense that a healthy sex life, combined with emotional intimacy, would be beneficial. Since humans are more advanced than the preying mantis and the female members of our species do not eat the male members after intercourse, but would rather keep them around, sex reinforces companionship. Studies have long shown that loneliness or the loss of a partner are detrimental to health. Married people live longer than those who are single. The emotional closeness couples share after a lifetime together explains the common finding that, after the first spouse dies, the second is rarely far behind.

Physiologically it would make sense that sex would be healthy as well, at least for men. Why? It is felt that the longer any carcinogens present in the body are in contact with a surface, the more likely they are to do their damage. Consider that increased water intake appears to lower the risk of bladder cancer by increasing urination and leaving less time for any carcinogens in the bladder to do their nasty deed. Likewise, more rapid transit time through the colon seems to protect against colon cancer, and colon cancer is almost unheard of in some tribes in Africa with diets that generate this. It would seem more frequent ejaculation could have a similar effect.

Should it stand to reason that what appears to be good for men should also be good for women? A few studies have supported this thought, although surprisingly few studies have been done. Postmenopausal women and women with children were left out in the studies, but sexual activity appears to protect against breast cancer in premenopausal women without children (Murrell, 1995). A few mechanisms were theorized. When women have an orgasm, a large amount of the hormone oxytocin is released, and it appears oxytocin has a protective effect against breast cancer. Oxytocin is also released with nipple stimulation. Interestingly, the reduction in risk was better for women who used non-barrier methods of contraception and it is possible that semen plays a role in cancer prevention in women.

For men, the scientific news may be good as well. Although breast cancer is less common in men than in women, one out of every one-hundred cases of breast cancer occurs in men. A study conducted in Greece revealed an inverse relationship between the frequency of orgasm during adulthood in men, and their risk of developing breast cancer (Petridou, 2000). While older studies had shown an increase in prostate cancer in men who were more active sexually, a more recent study out of Harvard did not see any increase. In this study, there was, in fact, a modest decrease in the incidence of prostate cancer in the men with the most activity (Leitzmann, 2004). The answer to the question smoldering in the mind of any man reading this book is this: the magic number necessary for reducing cases of cancer in this study is fifteen ejaculations per month!

Family Planning

"Have children while your parents are still young enough to take care of them."
—Rita Rudner

All other factors equal, and within reason, consider having children at a young age if possible. Giving birth to a first child before the age of thirty reduces the risk of developing breast cancer. The use of oral contraceptives to prevent pregnancy is discussed further in the section on medical treatment. Oral contraceptive use increases the risk of developing breast cancer in women under the age of thirty-five who have used birth control pills for at least six months, and poses a slightly increased risk of developing cervical cancer. On the up side, the long-term use of oral contraceptives has been linked with a decreased risk of developing ovarian cancer.

There has been controversy in the past about the role of elective abortion in contributing to the rise in breast cancer. This theory was based on the fact that, during the first trimester of pregnancy, many new breast cells are produced, and when pregnancy goes to term, breast cells stop their rapid growth. Concern was raised that elective abortion or miscarriage could disrupt this natural progression and, in the absence of a check on the multiplying cells based on changes at the end of pregnancy, malignancy could develop. In 2003, the National Cancer Institute (NCI) held a workshop regarding reproduction and breast cancer. They concluded that elective abortion and miscarriage do **not** increase the risk of developing breast cancer.

BREASTFEEDING

If it is possible and you are otherwise healthy, breastfeed your children for the first year of their lives. In addition to other known benefits, breastfeeding decreases the risk of the nursing mother developing breast and ovarian cancer, and decreases the risk of her breastfed children under the age of 15 developing cancer. Studies have shown that formula-fed children are much more likely to develop cancer than children who are breastfed more than six months (Bener, 2002; Smulevich, 1999; Kwan, 2004). Breastfeeding can also protect infants against infection with *H. pylori*, the leading cause of stomach cancer.

We offer a word of support here for mothers who are unable to, or choose not to, breastfeed. Childhood cancer is quite rare and though these statistics are alarming, we are dealing with small numbers. One of the authors worked with many wonderful, adoring mothers who did not breastfeed their infants, whether for reasons of inability, choice, or adoption. Our recommendation if you fall in this category would be to not "stress out" about bottle-feeding (stress damages your immune system). Instead, concentrate on the advantages bottle-feeding held/holds for you, such as allowing daddy more time to feed baby and having increased energy to play with your baby.

Practical Points

- ❑ Do not smoke in any form (cigarettes, cigars, or pipes) or use chewing tobacco.
- ❑ Avoid secondhand smoke.
- ❑ Maintain a body mass index less than or equal to twenty-five; do not gain more than 5 kg (11 lbs) in adulthood.
- ❑ Exercise in some way at least thirty minutes per day, ideally at least forty-five minutes per day.
- ❑ Children and adolescents should exercise at least sixty minutes per day.
- ❑ If you are a man, limit your alcohol intake to two drinks per day; women should limit intake to one drink per day.
- ❑ Develop ways to deal with stress in your life, whether it be yoga, prayer, meditation…
- ❑ Try to average getting around seven hours of sleep per night.
- ❑ Always sleep with the lights out.
- ❑ If possible, consider having children at an earlier age.
- ❑ For mothers, breastfeed if possible for at least six months.

Resources and Further Online Information

American Cancer Society's Guide to Quitting Smoking
www.cancer.org.

This American Cancer Society (ACS) Web site on smoking is very thorough, discussing addiction and the modalities available to make quitting more successful. The ACS also provides a quit line program. You can call 1-800-ACS-2345 to find a program in your area.

Smokefree.gov. You Can Quit Smoking Now!
www.smokefree.gov or 1-800-QUIT-NOW

Smokefree.gov is an online guide to quitting smoking complete with an evaluation of your unique situation. This site provides instant messaging and telephone support to assist those motivated to quit smoking.

CDC Tobacco Information and Prevention Source (TIPS) How to Quit
www.cdc.gov/tobacco/how2quit.htm.

This Web site provides many useful resources for quitting smoking in a positive fashion, stressing the benefits of not smoking.

NSTEP National Spit Tobacco Education Program. Smokeless Does NOT Mean Harmless
www.nstep.org.

NSTEP provides information on chewing tobacco with steps to assist in quitting.

Nutrition.gov. Smart Nutrition Starts here
www.nutrition.gov.

Nutrition.gov is an excellent site providing a wealth of information for achieving long-term weight control.

Weight Watchers
www.weightwatchers.com.

This Web site has information on the Weight Watchers program, and also provides recipes, information about fitness, and motivation plans for weight loss. A free online newsletter is available with many tips for weight loss.

National Center for Complimentary and Alternative Medicine. National Institute of Health. Back Grounder. Mind-Body Medicine. An Overview
www.nccam.nih.gov/health/backgrounds/mindbody.htm.

This Web site provides a definition of mind-body medicine, and discusses activities such as meditation and relaxation.

Worldwide Cancer Prayer Day
www.cancerprayerday.org.

Information on cancer and how to pray is presented on this site.

The President's Challenge Physical Activity and Fitness Awards Program
www.presidentschallenge.org/pdf/active_lifestyle.pdf.

Information on the Presidential Active Lifestyle Award offered for adults is discussed on this site; order forms are available for downloading for those who are interested.

Mayoclinic.com. Tools for Healthier Lives. Fitness
www.mayoclinic.com/health/fitness/SM99999

Mayoclinic.com reviews the benefits of exercise and offers tips about how to begin an exercise program. Information on sports nutrition and injury prevention is also provided.

Alcoholics Anonymous (AA)
www.alcoholics-anonymous.org.

The AA Web site provides information about alcohol abuse, as well as links to services available in your area.

Medline Plus. Sleep Disorder
www.nlm.nih.gov/medlineplus/sleepdisorders.html.

This resource provided by the National Institute of Health includes an interactive patient education tutorial on sleep disorders. It also contains a directory of sleep centers and providers in your area, as well as several links to credible sources offering suggestions about healthy sleep.

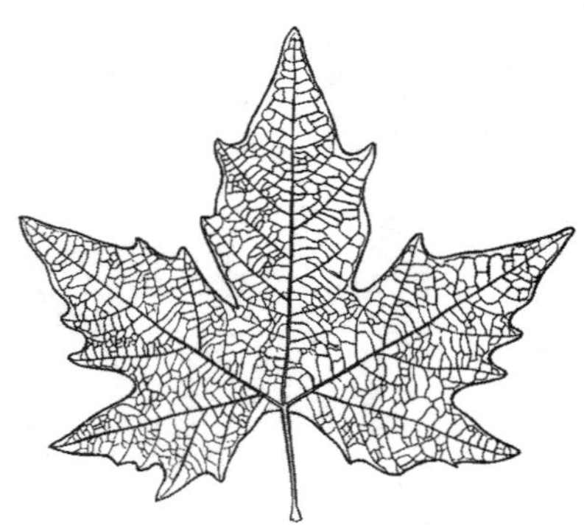

Chapter Seven

Medicine and Cancer Prevention

"Declare the past, diagnose the present, foretell the future: practice these acts. As to diseases, make a habit of two things – to help, or at least to do no harm."

—Hippocrates

We ask the reader to interpret this topic, of all the topics addressed in this book, with the most caution. Modern medicine has made great advances. We hesitate putting forth concerns regarding the evaluation and treatment of medical problems lest the reader consider "throwing the baby out with the bathwater" and lose perspective. All of life requires us to weigh the risks and benefits of options. That we have a number of options now is wonderful, but with more options come more personal decisions, and technology has offered us many.

Fifty years ago, physicians had limited options and the span of medicine was smaller. We did not have the wide array of prescription drugs, radiological procedures, and genetic tests at our disposal. As physicians are faced with an ever-increasing amount of data to consider, with less time to evaluate this with individual patients, consumers are being called on to take more active roles in their care.

This chapter will review some of the medications and procedures that have posed some concern from a cancer prevention standpoint. In many cases, the need for medication or radiological procedures far outweighs any risk posed by the treatment and should not be a cause for alarm. We wish to reinforce, however, that sometimes several options exist. We hope to give you a few basics to help you discuss these with your healthcare provider so that you both can make an informed decision regarding your care. We will then review some of the medical conditions that can predispose a person to developing cancer and discuss the role of family history in cancer.

MEDICATIONS

"Nearly all men die of their medicines, not of their diseases."

—Molière

Over 3 billion prescriptions for medications are given in the United States each year. Many of these have greatly improved the well-being of many people. Some can reduce the risk of stroke and heart disease. Some can even decrease the risk of developing cancer. Including non-prescription medications, and the recent explosion of nutritional supplements, the number of medicinal preparations we have access to is astronomical.

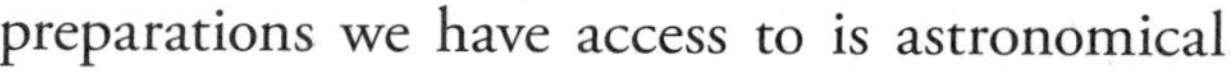

Prescription medications are subjected to intensive study before they are released to the masses, but even in this case, rare reactions and side effects may not be seen for some time. Nutritional supplements are not tested to the same degree, since they are not medications per se, but several have biochemical mechanisms and actions resembling those of prescription medications. It would be impossible to study every combination of prescription medications, over-the-counter medications, and nutritional supplements available, and we frequently only hear about possible interactions after several anecdotal reports. On top of this, the combination of these substances may have very different effects and side effects in different individuals depending on age, sex, body type, diet, and medical history.

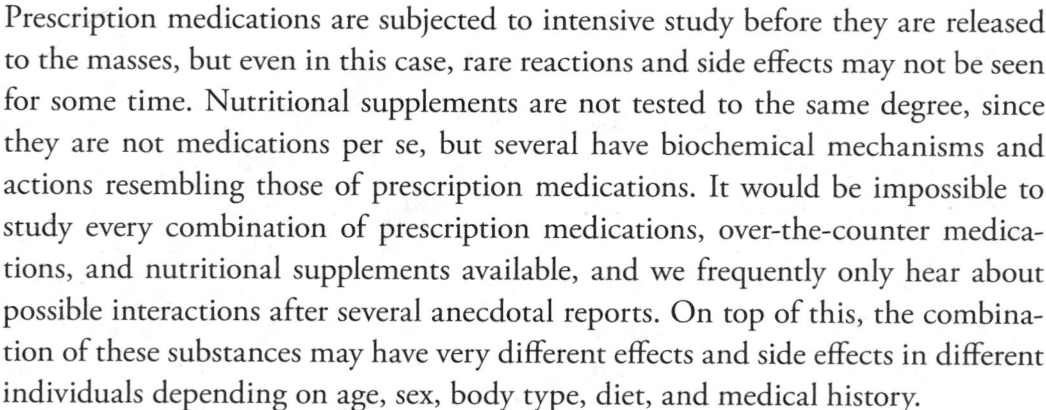

To emphasize the general importance of practicing discernment in evaluating your prescription and non-prescription choices, consider that the estimated cost of problems linked to medication use in an outpatient setting in the United States exceeded 177 billion in the year 2000! From 1969 until 2002, adverse reports submitted to the FDA's surveillance base on the roughly 6000 marketed drugs during that time amounted to 2.3 million cases. During that time, seventy-five prescription medications were withdrawn from the market, and several more restricted. With this information in mind, as well as concerns discussed below, consider four major questions when discussing medications with your healthcare provider and choosing over-the-counter products and supplements:

- What is the indication? What exactly is being treated?
- What is the necessity? Will using a medication or supplement lower your risk of developing a disease state or bring significant relief from a symptom? Would the ailment or symptom resolve on its own in time without treatment?
- What are possible alternatives? Is there a medication that may have fewer side effects? Would another alternative such as physical therapy work as well?
- What are possible interactions? It is important to bring all medications, including over-the-counter and nutritional supplements, with you to each appointment with your healthcare provider so that you can discuss how to lower your risk of interactions.

Unnecessary antibiotics

In 2004, the medical world was shaken a bit when scientists found a link between the incidence of breast cancer and antibiotic use. In this well publicized study put out by *The Journal of the American Medical Association*, it was found that women treated with more prescriptions of antibiotics had an increased risk of developing breast cancer, and that the risk increased further with greater duration of use (Velicer, 2005). There has been much debate about this study, but given the increasing resistance of microbes to antibiotics, it generates further concern over the overuse of antibiotics in the United States. A significant percent of antibiotics prescribed are for symptoms attributable to viruses. Antibiotics in general have absolutely no effect on viruses (there are a few anti-virals available that are used in very specific settings, but here we are discussing anti-bacterial antibiotics). In addition to this possible link with cancer, allergic reactions are not uncommon with many antibiotics and some can be very serious. The bottom line is to use antibiotics appropriately and only when necessary for an infection that is clearly thought to be bacterial, as determined by your healthcare provider.

It is also important to discard any leftover antibiotics when you are finished with them. Having leftover antibiotics available in your medicine cabinet raises the chance that, in your frustration over the symptoms of a viral infection, you will take some, hoping to alleviate the infection. However this will be to no avail and possibly to your detriment. Some infections, such as strep throat, that are not treated with a complete course of antibiotics can increase the risk of later developing rheumatic fever. Partial treatment with an inadequate dose or duration of antibiotics also increases the development of resistant strains of bacteria, since the bacteria present are not completely destroyed and are given the time to "get smart" and mutate, and subsequently become "immune" to the antibiotic in the future.

Metronidazole

Bacterial vaginosis is a common vaginal infection in women, diagnosed more frequently than yeast vaginitis. It is primarily a "nuisance infection," characterized by vaginal drainage and a fish-like odor. One of the primary treatments for this infection is the drug metronidazole, which is listed under California's proposition 65 as a chemical believed to cause cancer in humans (see Appendix C). While it may be necessary to use this to resolve your symptoms, make sure you consider the alternatives. There is an alternative antibiotic available, clindamycin, as well as natural remedies aimed at restoring the normal bacteria content of the vagina, that have been effective in many people.

Spironolactone

Spironolactone (Aldactone®) is another medication listed under California's Proposition 65. In most situations, the benefits of this medication would clearly outweigh its risks. It is used for treating fluid retention in cirrhosis of the liver, in heart failure, and in the treatment of primary aldosteronism. This medication is also used for non-life threatening disorders such as hirsutism (excess hair growth on womens' faces). In cases such as this, tweezing or waxing may be safer alternatives.

Oral contraceptives

Evaluate your birth control method carefully, keeping in mind your family history and other risk factors. The National Cancer Institute (NCI) sites a slight increase in the risk of developing cervical cancer and an increased risk of developing breast cancer in women under the age of thirty-five who had used birth control pills for at least six months. With long-term use, however, the use of oral contraceptives has been linked with a decreased risk of developing ovarian cancer.

Hormone replacement therapy (HRT)

Despite the widespread acceptance and praise of benefits it received a decade ago, postmenopausal estrogen therapy has now been named a known human carcinogen by the International Agency for Research on Cancer (IARC). Studies have shown an increase in the incidence of breast cancer in women exposed to combination estrogen-progestin replacement therapy. The breast cancers diagnosed in women who had used hormone replacement therapy were also larger and at more advanced stages when diagnosed.

Discuss alternatives to HRT with your healthcare provider if your menopausal symptoms are bothersome. He or she may be able to help you with dietary and activity recommendations to alleviate some discomfort. Several nutraceutical products such as black cohosh are now available, but studies to evaluate the efficacy and safety of such substances are lagging behind their use. Medications other than hormones are being used to help with some symptoms on occasion, but have their own side effects. Some physicians are working with bioidentical hormones, checking into whether the primary deficiency is in estrogen, progesterone, or other hormones, and then tailoring a woman's regimen based on specific symptoms and results from lab tests. Many of these include forms of estrogen and progesterone with more similarity to those produced naturally in the human body (versus some standard prescriptions), but the long-term effects are still unknown.

Some people continue to use HRT because of menopause's disabling symptoms. If you are using HRT, talk with your healthcare provider to make sure you are on the lowest dose possible that will manage your symptoms, and use the medications for the shortest amount of time possible. With your doctors supervision, consider drug holidays (periods of time when you do not take your medication) periodically to see if you continue to require it.

There is a lot of controversy about the management of menopausal symptoms. If you have symptoms that are affecting your well-being, we recommend you find a healthcare provider with a passion for working with menopausal women. Someone who has researched both traditional and alternative treatments, and has experience working with many menopausal women, may have increased insight into what will be most effective for you.

Anabolic steroids

Anabolic steroids should be used only when there are clear medical indications. The use of anabolic steroids for recreational purposes by men, such as to build muscle and improve athletic performance, can cause many complications. They have also been cited as probable human carcinogens. It has been noted repeatedly in studies that higher testosterone levels in men are associated with an increased risk of developing prostate cancer. This is disturbing considering the statistics regarding steroid use in the United States. A nationwide study of students in private and public high schools found that 6.6 percent of twelfth-grade male students had used anabolic steroids (Buckley, 1998). Only 21 percent of these students claimed to have received the drugs from a healthcare professional. Perhaps, in our cancer phobic society, educating our teenage boys that "steroids" are a carcinogen may help deter their desire to use these. Legitimate medical indications for use of anabolic steroids include wasting, associated with chronic diseases such as AIDS, some forms of infertility, and on occasion delayed puberty, **not** the desire to look like Mr. America or to bulk up for sports.

Methylphenidate

Methylphenidate (Ritalin®, Metadate CD®, Concerta®, others) has been the most widely used medication for attention deficit hyperactivity disorder (ADHD) in children and has been available for over fifty years. The diagnosis of ADHD in children has risen tremendously and sales of methylphenidate alone rose 500 percent from 1991 to 1999. Despite its widespread use, amazingly few studies have looked at long-term safety issues. One study on mice showed an increase in liver tumors but this was not shown in other animal studies (Dunnick, 1995). In 2005, a small sample of twelve children was evaluated with blood draws before and three months after starting therapy. Alarmingly all twelve children had a three-fold increase in chromosomal abnormalities and breakage (El-Zein, 2005). Higher chromosome abnormalities and breakage are associated with an increased risk of developing cancer later in life. This is a small sample size, we do not know if any of the abnormalities will return to normal, and, though chromosomal damage can be a precursor to cancer, none of these children may get cancer. What the study does accomplish is add a possible risk factor of developing cancer into the equation of risks versus benefits of treatment.

Before considering medications, we may want to look at what people did before prescriptions for ADHD skyrocketed. Sometimes changes in children's diets can make a significant difference in behavior. Perhaps they need a different structure to their activities. Is boredom in the exceptionally bright child, or frustration in another, presenting itself as hyperactivity or lack of concentration? Perhaps as parents, we need to alter **our** activities to accommodate our child's unique personality! Every child is different. We have seen children (and therefore parents and teachers as well) who have clearly benefited from prescription treatment for ADHD, but have seen many children for whom another intervention may have been more appropriate and safer. Weigh the risks and benefits of medications with your healthcare provider as part of a thorough evaluation of what is best for your child.

Medications for head lice

Studies have shown an association between the use of medications to treat head lice and the development of acute leukemia in children, with those exposed having double the risk (Menegaux, 2006). The highest risk appears to be with organochlorine based lice treatments such as lindane (Kwell®). Lindane is a potent animal carcinogen and has also been implicated as a cause of brain cancer in children. This risk is followed closely by that of pyrethroid-based treatments (Nix®, Rid®, others). The lowest risk was associated with organophosphorous-based products (Ovide®).

If it is necessary to treat your child with one of the available prescription or nonprescription medications, keep a few considerations in mind. Medications can be absorbed through the skin and a fair amount of chemical is absorbed with each application. Using extra medicine over that recommended on the label or prescription will not clear the infestation any faster, and treating family members who are unaffected will not help. Do not use the same medication more than two times if it does not work. Increasing resistance to head lice medication is emerging, and lack of improvement most likely indicates a change in medication is in order. Prevention is the best measure. Instruct your child not to share hats, hair accessories, brushes, or combs.

Iron supplements

Men and postmenopausal women rarely require supplemental iron, and the use of iron supplements could actually be dangerous. Iron increases the production of free radicals and higher blood levels of iron are associated with an increased risk of developing cancer. This increase was more than doubled when combined with high cholesterol levels (Mainous, 2005). Men and postmenopausal women should also choose multivitamins without iron for this reason. Iron supplements can also be dangerous for the one out of two hundred individuals who have the genetic disorder hemochromatosis, many of whom are unaware they carry the defect. Those with hemochromatosis have elevated blood levels of iron, which the body stores in the liver (sometimes leading to cirrhosis and even liver cancer) and the heart (leading to heart disease). Supplementation could further exacerbate this condition.

There are indications for iron supplements in men and postmenopausal women, such as certain forms of anemia where blood levels of iron are too low. We recommend using supplements only under the direction of your healthcare provider. If you are tired and concerned about anemia, make an appointment with your healthcare provider to be evaluated. There are many conditions that cause fatigue, and if anemia is diagnosed in men or postmenopausal women, further workup is needed to determine the cause.

Dietary Supplements

"Live in each season as it passes, breathe the air, drink the drink, taste the fruit and resign yourself to the influences of each. Let them be your only diet drink and botanical medicines."

—Henry David Thoreau

Since dietary supplements were allowed unrestricted reign in the over-the-counter market in 1994, there has been an exponential increase in the number of individuals who use these. While the authors have heard many anecdotes of wonderful results from using various preparations, we recommend finding out as much information as you can before using these. Choose dietary supplements wisely, ideally with the help of your physician, natural healthcare provider, or nutritionist.

A high intake of flavonoids, such as polyphenols and quercetin, is linked to lower rates of stomach, pancreatic, and lung cancer, and taking a supplement such as the flavonoid genistein may offer some protection against breast and prostate cancer. Recent studies have shown, however, that taking antioxidants such as flavonoids can decrease the effectiveness of chemotherapy and radiation for some cancers if taken at the same time.

One supplement, aristolochic acid, is a potent human carcinogen. Despite a 2001 FDA warning to consumers and industry, the authors were able to find this available through online pharmacies, and people likely still have bottles of supplements containing this ingredient in their medicine cabinets. Aristolochic acid is currently banned through much of Europe, in Japan, New Zealand, and Egypt and in part of South America.

Aristolochic acid has been marketed for treating premenstrual syndrome (PMS), to relieve menstrual cramps, for weight loss, and for gastrointestinal disorders. Unfortunately, it is also marketed under other names and is an ingredient in many combination remedies, making it more difficult to know if a supplement contains it. Aristolochic acid is also known as snakeroot, wild ginger, snakeweed, asarum, sangrel, sangree root, and serpentary. It can be a substitute for akebia, clematic, cocculus, Stephanie, and vladimiria. It can be found in Chinese herbal formulations including guang fangil, fang chi, mu xiang, ma dou ling, mu tong, and the Japanese formulations Kan-Mokutsu and Mokutsu.

There seems to be a general sense that nutritional supplements are safe. As noted above, this is not necessarily true, and supplements should be evaluated as should any medication you introduce to your body. When choosing supplements, the terms "herbal" and "natural" do not insure safety. Hemlock is "herbal" and "natural," but when Romeo and Juliet used it to commit suicide, it certainly did not enhance their love life!

Cancer Medications and Treatment

While many chemotherapy drugs are listed as carcinogens and many radiation and chemotherapy options could increase your risk of developing other cancers down the line, it is obvious that the benefits far outweigh theoretical risks in the majority of cases. In our current predicament where the five-year survival for cancers overall is only around 50 percent, no one should draw back from potentially curative therapy simply because of future risk. We should, however, be aware of all options, benefits, and long-term risks.

For example, women with breast cancer are often told the cure rate is similar whether they undergo a mastectomy or a lumpectomy with radiation. "Breast-conserving" surgery is widely praised. Our patients have told us that they failed to hear about the increased risk of developing other cancers (for example, lymphomas) down the line in women exposed to radiation to their chests. While this would probably not be a concern for an eighty-year-old woman diagnosed with breast cancer, and although other factors such as body image and emotional health cannot be understated, younger women should carefully discuss short-term and long-term risks and benefits of all options with their physician so they can make informed decisions.

Radiology

"My main frustration is the fear of cancer from low-dose radiation, even by radiologists."

—John Cameron

The discovery that radiation in the X-ray spectrum could diagnose internal problems from broken bones to head injuries brought dramatic advances to a science previously limited to listening to and examining a patient. Fractures could now be diagnosed and distinguished from abnormalities affecting tendons and ligaments. Once the fracture was diagnosed, there was a method of making sure it was corrected properly. Physicians in practice today cannot imagine **not** having this technology available. The last few decades have brought further advances with the introduction of imaging techniques from magnetic resonance imaging (MRI) to PET scans. With advances in the field of radiology, the spectrum of diseases diagnosed and treated with the available modalities has also expanded. In addition, as a science that was once used primarily to evaluate disorders that had clinical symptoms, medicine can now use radiological tests to screen for disease in patients with no symptoms. Before addressing possible concerns and questions to ask when you find yourself in the radiology department, it is important to have a little understanding of the three major radiological screening methods employed for detecting disease. New technologies are advancing rapidly but a review of other methods is beyond the scope of this book.

X-RAY

X-ray procedures, from the "plain" X-rays done in the clinic setting to extensive CT scans, involve radiation in the X-ray spectrum. In general, X-ray methods remain the best way to evaluate bones and look for bleeding in the brain. Any X-ray procedure involves some radiation exposure and carries a small risk of causing cancer, which is usually negligible relative to the condition for which the test is being performed. This method does cause concern, however, for pregnant women, where the use of diagnostic X-rays has been shown to increase the risk of these unborn children later developing leukemia and other cancers. Other concerns are discussed later in this chapter.

MRI

Magnetic resonance imaging uses magnetic energy and radio waves instead of X-rays to create images of the inside of the body. It is the preferred technique for looking for soft tissue disorders, such as disc disease, torn ligaments, and some forms of cancer. When used for breast imaging, it can also detect some abnormalities that may not be seen on mammograms. MRI is generally considered safe since there is no X-ray exposure; however, the magnets could dislodge and move any metal in the body (such as aneurysm clips, pacemakers, and shrapnel) and the possibility of this is routinely considered carefully before the procedure is performed. There is no known risk of MRI to pregnancy, but the procedure is still young. It is best to avoid MRI when pregnant if possible, but is most likely safer than X-ray procedures such as CT scans.

ULTRASOUND

Ultrasound is a procedure that bounces sound waves off organs and tissues and translates the information into pictures. No ionizing radiation is involved and ultrasound is generally considered safe during pregnancy. It is the preferred method for evaluating the fetus in pregnant women, and for looking for disorders such as ovarian cysts and gallbladder disease. It can also distinguish whether breast lumps that are palpated or seen on mammogram are solid or cysts.

GENERAL RADIOLOGY PRECAUTIONS

Since any diagnostic X-ray carries a small but finite risk of elevating your cancer risk, we offer a few questions to contemplate if you or your children require a diagnostic X-ray.

- Could another diagnostic method, for example ultrasound, MRI, lab test, or clinical exam, provide the same information without radiation? If not, what are the risks versus the benefits of waiting a few days? For women of childbearing age, could you wait until the first two weeks of your period to insure you are not pregnant?
- Is a competent lab technician performing the X-ray test? Underexposure and overexposure occur in clinical practice, resulting in unnecessary retakes, and consequently, excess radiation exposure.
- Is the X-ray facility up to date? Dates of inspection should be clearly marked.

RADIOLOGY PROCEDURES FOR CHILDREN

Recently, increasing concern has been raised about exposure of our children to medical radiation, particularly that present in CT scans. No known dose of radiation is completely safe for children, or for adults for that matter. Data from atomic bomb survivors has demonstrated a small but significant increase in cancer risk even in the doses used for pediatric CT scans (Brenner, 2001). Even the amount of radiation in a simple chest X-ray can have lasting consequences in children. Girls that carry a certain genetic predisposition to breast cancer are more than four times as likely to develop breast cancer in the future if they are exposed to chest X-rays before the age of twenty (Andrieu, 2006).

There are two unique considerations for radiation exposure in children put forth by the National Cancer Institute. As demonstrated in epidemiological studies, children are considerably more sensitive to radiation than are adults. Children also have a longer life expectancy and therefore more opportunity to exhibit the consequences of radiation damage. In 2002, the National Cancer Institute and the Society for Pediatric Radiology issued a guide for 160,000 physicians asking them to take measures to avoid children's exposure to CT scan radiation. In this guide, they asked physicians to:

- Perform only necessary CT scans.
- Adjust exposure parameters based on the child's size and weight and the specific area of the body to be scanned.
- Minimize the use of multiple scans, which result in considerable increases in radiation doses.

Since most CT scanners do not adjust dosages automatically, it is imperative that parents be informed consumers and talk to their physicians about lower CT doses. While it is no guarantee, choosing a facility that caters to children, ideally with pediatric radiologists on staff, may eliminate some of this burden on parents.

Radiation as a Screen for Disease

As the public becomes more health conscious and recognizes more and more the limitations of the physician's eyes and ears during a clinical exam, we have turned to the laboratory and radiology department to offer guidance. Many a patient has questioned us and inquired about a lab test or X-ray that could detect hidden, yet-to-manifest-itself disease. In the twenty-first century, some of this technology has reared its head for better or for worse. For a mere $900 to $1500 you can have a total body CAT scan designed to try to detect previously unknown tumors lying anywhere in your body. Nevertheless, cost is not everything.

Elective full-body CT scans have been promoted recently in the United States as a way to search for and find hidden diseases at an early and hopefully curable stage. The authors have witnessed the excitement of individuals having this done! In a national telephone interview published in *The Journal of the American Medical Association (JAMA)*, 73 percent of respondents stated they would prefer a total-body CT scan instead of receiving $1,000 in cash (Schwartz, 2004). Unfortunately, there is no evidence that whole-body CT is effective in detecting any disease early enough to prolong life. On top of this is the risk from the radiation itself. It has been estimated that the risk of dying from cancer induced by radiation is 0.08

percent from one total body CT scan (Brenner, 2004). The results of radiation are cumulative, and add up with each subsequent scan, so using this as a surveillance technique increases the risk further.

To understand the significance of this, compare the radiation from a body scan to that experienced by atomic bomb survivors, in whom exposure has clearly been documented to increase cancer risk. In a typical full-body CT scan, patients are exposed to a radiation dose equivalent to that received by some survivors of the Hiroshima and Nagasaki atomic bombs. During a full-body CT scan the body absorbs roughly 13 milliSieverts of radiation. This is equivalent to the dose absorbed by people living 2.4 km from the center of the atomic blasts! The FDA has advised against the practice of recommending full-body CT scans to screen for disease in healthy patients.

We advise that if you are concerned about underlying disease, have a long talk with your healthcare provider. If you have behaviors that are causing you concern, address them. If you smoke, quit. If you have questions about your diet, read this book carefully, and then find a good nutritionist to help you incorporate five to nine servings of fruits and vegetables per day into your diet and to guide you toward healthy, not unhealthy, food choices. If you are concerned about exposures at work, take measures to make sure you are protected adequately. Finding a disease early does not guarantee a cure, and there has been controversy with some cancer types about whether picking up a cancer early really increases life expectancy; the patient may have lived longer just because he or she was diagnosed sooner. For now, we believe early detection makes a difference and clearly does with several cancer types, but the reader should be cautioned to "first of all do no harm" to themselves, as more tests such as full-body CT scans are likely to be presented as options in the future.

Our knowledge of the information needed to screen for cancer, in light of the risk posed by radiation, is continually changing, and can be illustrated by changes in screening smokers for lung cancer. Until fairly recently, smokers were typically given screening chest X-rays when they went in for a physical to screen for cancer, and many people appear surprised that this is no longer done. Studies have now shown that routine X-rays do not pick up lung cancers in smokers any sooner than they would have been detected by symptoms alone, and consequently do not improve survival. Screening X-rays in the presence of this information would only be expected to increase the risk of cancer to some degree from repeated X-ray exposures. If you are a smoker and looking for screening, the only test that has been shown to pick up lung cancer at an earlier stage than symptoms alone would reveal is the CT scan. A limited, spiral CT scan of the chest to screen for lung cancer is usually an out-of-pocket expense not covered by insurance. If you are concerned enough to invest in the test, go ahead, but consider putting your money into a good smoking-cessation program as well. Smoking causes many diseases beyond cancer.

Medical Conditions That May Predispose a Person to Developing Cancer

"The more serious the condition, the more important it is for you to fight back, mobilizing all your resources—spiritual, emotional, intellectual, physical."

—Norman Cousins

The following discussion is in no way a complete or exhaustive account of the many medical conditions that can predispose a person to develop cancer, but is put forth to educate and enlighten the layperson in a few areas as well as to illustrate the interaction of many individual factors in the development of cancer. Some diagnoses that raise the risk of developing cancer, such as cirrhosis from alcohol abuse or hepatitis B or C, are discussed elsewhere in this book. The issues presented span a wide array, from hereditary disorders to in-utero exposures to post-treatment concerns. Having a predisposition to develop cancer by whatever means does not mean you will develop cancer, as will be stated again later, and the reader should not feel pessimistic over the fate they were dealt. Our hope is that having an awareness of such risks will cause the reader to inquire further into their environmental exposures, lifestyle practices, and diet to tip the "multifactorial causes" as discussed in Chapter Three in their favor.

COLON POLYPS

Roughly one in twenty people will develop colorectal cancer in their lifetime, and 90 percent of cases should be preventable with proper screening. Unfortunately, only a small percentage of those at risk have undergone recommended screening and evaluation. The majority of colon cancers begin as benign polyps, non-cancerous growths that occur in the large intestine. Most polyps do not turn into cancer, and 30 to 50 percent of middle-aged and older adults will develop at least one polyp.

There are three major types of colon polyps with differing potential to become cancerous. **Hyperplastic** polyps rarely become cancerous. **Inflammatory** polyps are usually non-threatening as well, but tend to occur in people who suffer from inflammatory bowel diseases that do raise the risk of colon cancer. About 30 percent of polyps are **adenomatous** polyps that have the potential to become cancerous. These in turn are divided into tubular adenomatous polyps, and villous adenomatous polyps, the latter of which are less common but more likely to become malignant. Adenomatous polyps are unlikely to be cancerous when they are small, but with time and increasing size, the risk of them becoming malignant increases. In general, it takes at least five to ten years for an adenomatous polyp to regress to cancer, allowing a large window of opportunity for detection and removal.

Having a family history of colon cancer quadruples the risk you could develop this in the future, but in some cases the risk is even greater. Two major genetic syndromes carry a very high risk for the development of colorectal cancer. These gene mutations are inherited in an autosomal dominant fashion, so that if either of your parents carry the mutation there is a 50 percent chance you will inherit it. A rare disorder, **familial adenomatous polyposis,** is responsible for about 1 percent of colon cancer cases. People with this syndrome frequently have hundreds of polyps throughout their colons. Cancers usually develop beginning around age twenty and by age forty, nearly everyone who carries this mutation will have developed cancer if it has not been prevented by surgery. Up to 10 percent of colon cancers are secondary to **hereditary nonpolyposis colon cancer (Lynch's syndrome).**

Individuals with this syndrome do not have the hundreds of polyps seen in people with polyposis, but most develop colon cancer by the age of forty-five. Carriers of this mutation are also at high risk for developing other cancers, including those of the uterus, ovaries, stomach, small intestine, kidney, and bile duct. Taking a thorough family history will usually alert your healthcare provider to this syndrome, since a large number of people who are carriers have at least three relatives who have been diagnosed with colon cancer.

Most polyps do not cause any symptoms. If they do, common signs include rectal bleeding, dark stools, or anemia due to blood loss too small to be visualized. Rarely, polyps can become large and cause constipation, diarrhea, or pain secondary to obstruction.

It is currently recommended that all adults be screened for polyps and colon cancer beginning at age fifty, ideally with colonoscopy, which is the most accurate method of detection. In some cases, such as having a family history of colon cancer, or having a relative with the hereditary syndromes mentioned above, screening may be recommended much earlier.

DES EXPOSURE

DES (diethylstilbestrol) is a hormone that was used to decrease the risk of premature labor in pregnant women until it was discontinued in the early 1960s. Exposure to DES in utero raises the risk of developing cancer, specifically clear cell carcinoma of the vagina and cervix in female children born to mothers who were treated during pregnancy. Male children born to mothers treated with DES may have an increased risk of testicular cancer as well. Mothers who were treated with DES during pregnancy have an increased risk of later developing breast cancer. Women who were treated with DES should be vigilant about breast cancer screening recommendations. Women whose mothers took DES during pregnancy should have yearly pelvic exams and inform their healthcare providers of their exposure. Men whose mothers took DES should be taught how to perform self-testicular exams and should perform them regularly.

Gastroesophageal reflux disease (GERD)

Chronic gastroesophageal reflux (GERD) can damage the esophagus, ultimately leading to esophageal cancer. Inflammation of the esophagus occurs when the acid contents of the stomach flow back into the esophagus. The most common symptom is heartburn, but some people can experience difficulty swallowing, a chronic cough, chest pain, or no symptoms at all. A pre-cancerous condition, Barrett's esophagus, develops in approximately 10 to 20 percent of people with chronic GERD, and can be visualized during endoscopy. Of those people who develop Barrett's esophagus, 0.5 to 1 percent will develop esophageal cancer per year. Since esophageal cancer has a dismal prognosis, secondary prevention through screening for Barrett's esophagus offers an opportunity to be alert to its development early, and to take measures to decrease the damage from reflux. It has been recommended that anyone experiencing chronic GERD for a period of five or more years be screened with endoscopy.

If you experience heartburn regularly, discuss this with your healthcare provider. Some people consider this only a nuisance symptom but, as noted above, it can be of more concern. Many conservative measures can be taken to reduce the damage from reflux and to control symptoms. These include eating small meals more frequently, avoiding eating for three hours prior to lying down, raising the head of your bed six inches, and avoiding foods that make your symptoms worse, such as citrus foods, chocolate, alcohol, caffeine, and fatty foods. It is also beneficial to address issues that predispose a person to reflux, such as smoking and obesity. Several medications are available that can help when conservative measures fail, and in rare cases surgery is needed to correct the problem.

Undescended testicles in male children

Undescended testicles occur in approximately 3 to 4 percent of male infants at birth. Most cases resolve spontaneously, but surgical treatment may be required if testicles do not descend by one year of age. Undescended testicles that do not descend on their own significantly raise the risk of later developing testicular cancer, which is the leading kind of cancer at this time for men aged eighteen to forty. Surgery to repair testicles that do not descend spontaneously, while it may help preserve fertility, does not lower the subsequent risk of cancer. Thankfully, most cases of testicular cancer are very treatable and carry a very good long-term prognosis.

Boys and men who have a history of undescended testicles should be taught at a young age to perform self-testicular exams and have regular medical visits to screen for cancer. Many healthcare providers have shower cards available similar to the breast exam cards given to women. These cards provide instruction on performing self-exams and provide a visual reminder to do this frequently.

Inflammatory bowel disease

Ulcerative colitis, a medical condition involving inflammation of the colon, significantly increases the risk of developing colon cancer. About 5 percent of individuals with this condition will develop cancer, and therefore careful monitoring is imperative. Treatments to decrease inflammation or remove the affected portion of the colon, as well as dietary changes, may decrease the risk, but this is uncertain at this time. Screening for dysplasia (precancerous changes) is currently the standard of care.

Those individuals with involvement of the whole colon should begin getting screening colonoscopies eight years after diagnosis. Colonoscopies should be initiated fifteen years after diagnosis for those with involvement of only the left colon. Colonoscopies are then recommended every one to two years to screen for dysplasia. Symptoms associated with ulcerative colitis include abdominal pain and bloody diarrhea. Some patients also suffer from fatigue, anemia secondary to blood loss, weight loss, arthritis, and osteoporosis. Some other causes of inflammatory bowel disease, such as Crohn's disease, also increase the risk of developing colon cancer, and patients with these deserve special monitoring as well.

Hemochromatosis

Hemochromatosis, or "iron overload disease," is a genetic disorder with an incidence of one in two hundred people. One of the most common genetic disorders in the United States, it is transmitted in an autosomal recessive fashion. If you inherit the defective gene from both parents, you may develop the disease. If you inherit the gene from only one parent, you will become a carrier and may pass this on to your children but usually you will not have symptoms. The underlying problem in hemochromatosis is a disorder in iron metabolism that causes the body to absorb and store too much iron. Excess iron in these individuals is stored in the liver, pancreas, heart, and joints and can lead to cirrhosis of the liver, liver cancer, diabetes, and heart disease.

If you have any relatives with hemochromatosis, or that have suffered from cirrhosis or liver cancer but did not drink alcohol, have your iron level checked. Hemochromatosis is an under-diagnosed medical condition and many people are unaware they carry the defect until they develop complications or for some reason have their iron level checked for another reason. Men usually manifest symptoms between the ages of thirty and fifty, and women commonly do not show symptoms until after the age of fifty. The most common symptoms include joint pain, fatigue, abdominal pain, and a bronze appearance to the skin.

Medical treatment is available to those diagnosed with hemochromatosis to lower later risks. Phlebotomy (removing blood) is the primary treatment. For these people, avoiding other factors that may further raise their risk of liver disease and liver cancer, such as excess alcohol consumption and hepatitis infection, is very important.

Diabetes

In addition to its well-known complications such as heart disease, kidney problems, eye damage, and neuropathy, diabetes carries an increased risk of developing cancer. Type 2 diabetes is associated with an increased risk of developing colon (Larsson, 2005), uterine (Anderson, 2001), liver (Adami, 1996), breast (Weiderpass, 1999), and kidney (Lindbland, 1999) cancers, and non-Hodgkin's lymphoma (Cerhan, 1997). In an attempt to break through the pessimism for a moment, we point out that one study showed a lower risk of developing prostate cancer in patients with diabetes (Weiderpass, 2002). Type 1 diabetes is associated with an increased chance of developing stomach, cervix, and uterine cancers (Zendehdel, 2003). Preventing cancer is simply one more reason for diabetic patients to monitor their blood sugars carefully. At the clinical level, the authors have been somewhat surprised by how lightly the public addresses the diagnosis of diabetes and "pre-diabetes." Studies have shown that simply having the diagnosis of diabetes means a person is as likely to suffer a heart attack as someone who has already had a heart attack. This is a frightening figure for those individuals with diabetes and for society as a whole, since the number of people diagnosed with diabetes is expected to continue to increase, as our nation becomes progressively more obese.

H. PYLORI/PEPTIC ULCER DISEASE

Infection with *H. pylori* and this bacteria's role in peptic ulcer disease and gastric cancer is discussed in Chapter Five. If you have a history of peptic ulcer disease, make sure to read that section carefully and seek medical attention if you have not been evaluated or treated for *H. pylori*. *H. pylori* is currently considered the leading cause of stomach cancer worldwide.

CHILDHOOD RADIATION FOR MEDICAL CONDITIONS

Thanks to increased understanding of the risks of radiation, X-ray treatment is no longer used for minor medical conditions. Not that long ago, however, X-ray treatments were used for acne and to treat ringworm. If you were one of the patients treated in this way, let your physician know so he or she can screen you appropriately. Radiation to treat these minor conditions in childhood has been associated with an increased risk for developing thyroid and head and neck cancers.

Women who have received radiation therapy to their chest for another cancer (for example, Hodgkin's disease or non-Hodgkin's lymphoma) as children or young adults carry a significantly higher risk of developing breast cancer (up to twelve times the average risk). More involved screening, such as breast MRI for early detection, may want to be considered in addition to traditional screening.

BREAST IMPLANTS

While several studies have shown that breast implants do not affect the risk of developing breast cancer, having implants can make standard mammograms more difficult to interpret. If you have breast implants, make sure you discuss with your physician additional studies, such as implant displacement views, which can be ordered to see breast tissue more clearly. In a large study conducted by the National

Cancer Institute in 2000, breast cancers were detected at a somewhat more advanced stage in patients who had implants compared to non-implant patients. Despite a later stage of detection in the implant group, the mortality (death rate) of the implant and non-implant patients was the same (Brinton, 2000).

Breast implants were first marketed in the United States in 1962. There are two primary types available at this time. Both types involve a silicone sack, which is filled either with saline or silicone gel. The majority of implants at this time are the saline type. A word of caution is in order, despite the reassuring studies. Silicone implants can cause scar tissue to form, and scar tissue in the breast from other causes such as trauma has been correlated with breast cancer. In addition, one of the breakdown products of the polyurethane foam used in some implants in the past is 2,4 – toulenediamine (TDA). This was removed from hair dyes in 1971 after it was found to cause cancer, but continued to be used in breast implants. It is estimated that 110,000 women have silicone gel filled implants with this polyurethane coating (which was used to decrease the chance of rupture) and was discontinued in the manufacture of breast implants in 1991. The FDA evaluated this and felt it conferred a negligible risk and does not recommend prophylactic removal of implants containing this coating.

Family History of Cancer

"If you don't know [your family's] history, then you don't know anything. You are a leaf that doesn't know it is part of a tree."

—Michael Crichton

It is estimated that 10 percent of cancers have a genetic predisposition. Rather than regretting that you were born into the wrong family if you have relatives with cancer, let this be a positive note. If 10 percent of cancers have a genetic predisposition, then 90 percent of cancers have an environmental component that can be evaluated and possibly altered. Sometimes having a family history of cancer may even prove to be beneficial in a roundabout way by raising a person's awareness of his or her cancer risks. One of the authors used to encounter women who were quite concerned about their risk of developing breast cancer, given a positive family history. These women tended to be vigilant about doing self-breast exams, having mammograms, and eating well, all to lower their risk. Considering only 10 percent of breast cancer cases are felt to be hereditary, and one in seven women will be diagnosed with breast cancer in their lifetimes, a much larger number of women will develop breast cancer who do not carry this worry and may not be as motivated to undergo screening.

A predisposition does not mean a guarantee of cancer, just a tendency to develop this in a setting of other factors. As noted previously, cancer is a multifactorial disease. Some people may have a strong tendency to develop cancer based on their family histories, but, through wise choices in diet and lifestyle, beat the odds. Other individuals may have only a slight genetic tendency towards developing a certain cancer, but, given unhealthy aspects of their lifestyles, make themselves much more prone to develop that cancer.

The genetics of cancer can be somewhat confusing as well. Some cancers or syndromes have a very strong hereditary component or tendency to foster cancer (such as endocrine tumors like medullary carcinoma of the thyroid) and others only seem to run in families to a small degree. Some cancers do not seem to carry any genetic predisposition at all. Certain types of cancers, such as ovarian and breast cancers, tend to run together in families. Some families have a predisposition to cancer but it shows up as many different types of cancer in different individuals (cancer family syndromes).

Taking a thorough family history of cancer and relaying the information to your healthcare provider is an important part of your cancer prevention arsenal. We encourage readers to use the worksheets in the appendix and question their family members prior to their next appointment with their physicians. While certain cancers are more likely to have an inherited component, such as those of the breast, ovary, colon and prostate, as well as malignant melanoma, it is important to list all cancers, as new information is brought forth continually. Some cancers, such as pancreatic cancer, were considered primarily environmental in the past. It is now known that there is a genetic predisposition towards the development of pancreatic cancer, and screening techniques for those with a family history may come into play in the near future. Cancers that are considered uncommon should be noted and further information obtained if possible, since several rare tumor types may be part of a genetic syndrome. If any possible predisposing factors (such as asbestos exposure, smoking or alcoholism) are present in your family members, note this as well.

A complete family history of cancer should go beyond those family members diagnosed with cancer. Check to see if anyone in your family has been diagnosed with colon polyps, and if so, which type. If uncertain, ask your family members if they were adenomatous polyps (the type that can progress to cancer) or hyperplastic polyps. Ask if any family members have had abnormal Pap smears, suspicious findings on mammograms, abnormal PSAs, or abnormal skin lesions that are being "followed." Share your findings with them as well. None of us are completely aware of how we affect those around us in our everyday life, but asking a few questions and sharing your research could increase their knowledge and help protect them from cancer as well.

If you have a significant family history of cancer, find a healthcare provider who is up to date on the latest screening techniques and has an interest in prevention and early detection. Concerning issues in a family history include: several family members who have had cancer; more than two relatives with breast cancer or ovarian cancer; family members that have had more than one type of cancer; or a family history of any uncommon cancers. Genetic testing is available for certain situations, such as for breast and ovarian cancers. Early or additional screening and increased surveillance may be considered in some cases, for example, colonoscopy before the age of fifty for a person with a family history of colon cancer. If possible, find a healthcare provider who can guide you in dietary and environmental approaches to decrease your risk.

PRACTICAL POINTS

- ❑ Avoid unnecessary antibiotics.
- ❑ Understand the risks and benefits of medications you are taking and be aware of alternatives.
- ❑ Avoid hormone replacement therapy unless your symptoms are disabling. If you must use hormone replacement therapy, use the smallest dose possible for the least amount of time, monitored by a healthcare professional who is passionate about menopausal issues and aware of alternatives available.
- ❑ Practice caution and view dietary supplements as you would any medication.
- ❑ Do not use anabolic steroids to build muscle or increase athletic performance.
- ❑ If your child is diagnosed with ADHD, try conservative methods before resorting to medications.
- ❑ If you are a man or postmenopausal woman, do not use iron supplements or vitamins containing iron without the advice of your healthcare provider.
- ❑ If your child comes home with head lice, teach him or her prevention, request the safest medication possible, and do not use the same preparation more than two times if it is ineffective.
- ❑ Question any X-ray procedure you are having done with regard to safety and available alternatives.
- ❑ If your child requires a CT scan to diagnose a medical problem, ask if the exposure parameters have been adjusted to your child's size.

- ☐ Stay away from full-body CT scans to detect cancer if you are otherwise healthy and have no symptoms.
- ☐ If you have heartburn frequently, discuss this with your healthcare provider.
- ☐ If you or your mother was treated with DES during pregnancy, make sure your healthcare provider is aware of this.
- ☐ If your male child had an undescended testicle that persisted past his first birthday or was operated on, teach him the importance of self-testicular exams at a young age.
- ☐ Complete a thorough review of your family history of cancer and complete the worksheets in the appendix to share with your healthcare provider.
- ☐ Keep in mind that 80 to 95 percent of cancers have an environmental component: if you have a positive family history of cancer, there is still a lot you can do to raise your odds against developing cancer.

Resources and Further Online Information

FDA.com. Online Information Portal and Discussion Groups
www.fda.com

This Web site has a section on forums, links, and resources for consumers, with an extensive selection of topics and links regarding medications. In addition to providing drug specific information on the myriad of medications currently available, topics ranging from whole body CT scans to food allergies are addressed.

Medline Plus. Hemochromatosis
www.nlm.nih.gov/medlineplus/hemochromatosis.html.

The U.S. National Library of Medicine and the National Institute of Health provide this site, which contains an overview of hemochromatosis and information on current methods of diagnosis and treatment.

American Diabetes Association
www.diabetes.org/

The American Diabetes Association's Web site contributes a wide array on helpful information on diabetes, including tips on nutrition, weight loss, and exercise. Local events and information in your area can be accessed as well by zip code.

U.S. Department of Health and Human Services. U.S. Surgeon General's Family History Initiative
www.hhs.gov/familyhistory/

This site has an excellent section entitled "My Family Health Portrait" for creating a family history. You can also receive a free copy of "My Family Health Portrait" by calling 1-888-275-4772.

Genome.gov. National Human Genome Research Institute. National Institute of Health
http://genome.gov/health

This Web site provides information about genetic testing for specific cancers.

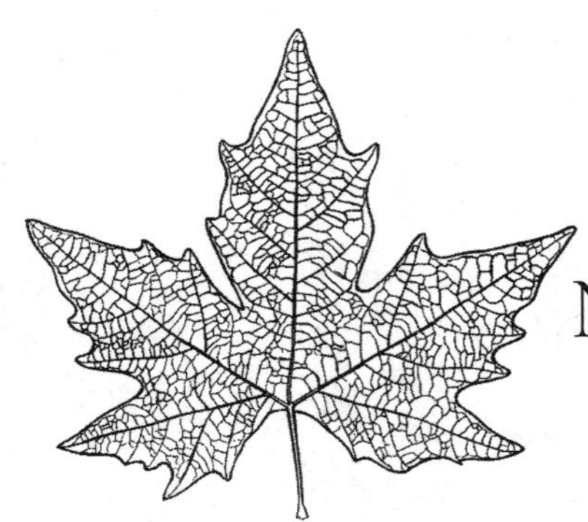

Chapter Eight

Nutrition and Cancer Prevention

"Let food be thy medicine and medicine be thy food."

—Hippocrates

"The junk food industry is peddling junk science."

—Bill Lockyer, Attorney General Of California

Imagine a machine with a trillion parts, each part undergoing changes twenty-four hours a day, seven days a week, with operating systems ranging from voice recognition to hydraulics to sewage systems, connected by wiring that could circumference the globe. Were you placed in charge of this machine, worth a mere few hundred thousand to the powers that be but priceless and totally irreplaceable, would you be careful to use the proper fuel?

The time-faded statement "You are what you eat" carries much truth. Lacking the chlorophyll plants have, we cannot stand still and obtain our energy from the sun. The remarkable food tablets common in science fiction decades ago have yet to become reality. Our bodies are remarkably designed machines, and what we eat is the fuel that either helps us run smoothly, or makes us cough and sputter and sometimes die. Considering this, and the fact that the typical American diet has an analogous octane level lower than we would allow in our cars, it is astonishing we do not "break down" more often.

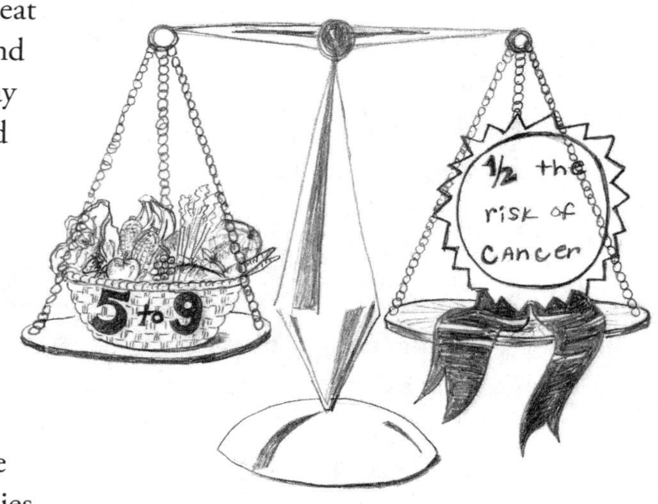

Controversy over what to eat abounds. "Fad" diets emerge and while the individual foods may have merit, isolating one food item to the exclusion of a balanced diet eventually leads to its rejection and replacement by the next miracle diet. An adequate amount of some foods and vitamins is good but, when eaten or taken in excess, can be dangerous. The recommendations of some studies have shifted 180 degrees over the last few decades. Controversy and 180-degree turns abound in medicine. In 1927, 10,000 physicians actually recommended smoking cigarettes for health! So how do we interpret the data? The conclusion of most studies end with a call for further studies—an honorable conclusion—but where does that leave us in our quest for knowledge about healthy foods and what to eat today?

Our number one recommendation is to consume a wide variety of foods. The principles behind this are the foundation of a cancer-prevention diet. Eat a variety of foods so you are more likely to receive an ample supply of the nutrients you need to stay healthy. Eat a variety of foods so you avoid repeated exposure to carcinogens that may be present in certain foods. Avoid diets that isolate and recommend excesses of certain foods. Avoid diets that eliminate foods, even if only for a few days or weeks, that are necessary for long-term health. Eating five to nine servings of fruits and vegetables a day, minimizing fast food, and choosing products less likely to be contaminated by hormones or pesticides should cover the bases, allowing a home run against most opposing carcinogen teams. For those extra sneaky carcinogens, adding a variety of "super-foods and nutrients" could be an additional week of spring training in your nutritional fitness program to prevent cancer.

5 TO 9

"I don't understand why asking people to eat a well-balanced vegetarian diet is considered drastic, while it is medically conservative to cut people open."

—Dean Ormish, M.D.

People who eat five or more servings of fruits and vegetables daily have only one-half the risk of developing cancer as do those who eat one or two servings a day. Sadly, the average American currently eats only one serving of fruit and one serving of vegetables per day. Many of our children express disgust over fruits and vegetables, but we cannot afford to wait until they "outgrow it" and develop a taste for these later in life. Childhood consumption of fruit lowers their risk of developing cancer before they reach adulthood. The regular intake of oranges, orange juice, and bananas in the first two years of life is correlated with a decreased risk of childhood leukemia in children ages 2 to 14 (Kwan, 2004). Eating fruit in childhood also lowers children's cancer risks later on when they become adults (Maynard, 2003).

Increasing dietary intake from an average of two up to nine servings of fruits and vegetables per day may seem formidable, so it is helpful to discuss what a serving size is. A serving is frequently smaller that most people realize, especially with our growing portion sizes in the U.S. A serving is defined as:

- 1 medium sized fruit
- ¾ cup (6 oz) of 100-percent fruit or vegetable juice
- 1 cup of raw leafy vegetables
- ½ cup cooked dry peas or beans
- ¼ cup dried fruit
- ½ cup cooked vegetables
- ½ cup cut-up fruits or vegetables

Many children, and some adults, are "picky" eaters, but a few ideas can help with even the fussiest. Become creative with ways to "hide" vegetables and fruits in the meals you prepare. Use sauces and dips if needed to add flavor. Remember, you can drink some of your fruits and vegetables, and make juices or smoothies. Also, keep in mind that you can develop a taste for foods you do not currently enjoy. Most smokers did not like the taste of their first cigarettes. Most alcoholics did not relish the taste of their first drinks. Most coffee lovers did not especially savor their first sips of coffee. Research on children has shown that if foods are frequently re-introduced in small amounts, many of them are accepted after ten to fifteen meals (Gallop, 2005).

Suggestions for Getting Five to Nine Servings of Fruits and Vegetables per Day

- Try juicing.
- Freeze seedless red grapes. Frozen red grapes have become one of the author's favorite desserts.
- A vegetable made more appetizing by dipping it in a small amount of dip is better than no vegetable at all.
- Add vegetables to lasagna, casseroles, and spaghetti.
- Add fruits to cereal; point out the pictures of fruit and cereal portrayed on cereal boxes to your children. It may raise their interest.
- Keep dried fruit in the car as a quick snack.
- Try caramel dip for apples.
- Grow a vegetable garden.
- Visit the farmer's market and try new vegetables; ask the vendors how to prepare these.
- Add blueberries to pancakes, muffins, and waffles.
- Snack on bean dip and salsa.
- Visit the apple orchard.
- Keep fresh fruit on the kitchen counter.
- Try different ethnic foods to learn new ways of preparing and flavoring vegetables.

- Keep cut-up vegetables (cucumbers, peppers, broccoli, cauliflower, celery, grape or cherry tomatoes, carrots, green onions) in the refrigerator and put out with each meal.
- Make soups with a variety of beans and vegetables.
- Freeze 100-percent juice as "popsicles."
- Involve children in shopping and challenge them to pick out new fruits and vegetables.
- Involve your children in planning a cancer-prevention diet. Contrary to what the typical adolescent reflects in their facial expressions, children ARE interested in health and DO hear what we talk about. If you share ideas regarding healthy food choices with them, they may remind you to buy fruits and veggies when you are racing through the grocery store or frantically stopping for fast food. Thus, we offer a word of caution: only do this if you are willing to listen to their reminders!
- Shop the periphery of the grocery store. For fun, try to purchase everything fresh and avoid the aisles.
- Go to the library, check your bookshelves, or go to the bookstore. Find cookbooks with pictures or search online for new ways to prepare fruits and vegetables.
- Try out vegetarian recipes.

If you simply do not like fruits and vegetables, could a pill do it? The answer is a clear no, at least in this moment of time with our expanding but still quite limited understanding of nutrition. There are over 900 types of phytochemicals that have been identified in fruits and vegetables that are associated with the prevention not only of cancer but of diabetes, heart disease, and high blood pressure. More await discovery. Several of the multitude of phytochemicals available probably work together in disease prevention. It would be difficult if not impossible to provide this in a tablet or drink, given our present state of knowledge.

The Fast Food Epidemic

"When you see the golden arches, you are probably on your way to the pearly gates."

—William Castelli, M.D.

Since White Castle opened its doors in 1921 selling hamburgers for five cents, the fast food industry has boomed: one fourth of Americans eat at a fast food restaurant every day. In our hurried lives, we praise the convenience and are pleased with the amount of food we can get for the money we spend. Many public schools and even hospitals have welcomed aboard this inexpensive time-saver. Since fast food provides the ready-at-hand sustenance that allows us to scurry about our busy lives, is there any reason to pass up this ease and return to the "antiquated" practice of preparing food in our homes? Is there any truth to the scenario portrayed in the 2004 film *Super-Size Me*?

The CARDIA study published in *Lancet* in 2005 gave a somber answer to this question. In this study of young adults, it was found that white people who eat fast food twice or more a week have a 50 percent greater risk of obesity than if they did not. The risk of developing abnormal glucose control, otherwise known as "prediabetes," was double compared to that of the non-fast food crowd. Combine this with two and a half hours per day of TV watching, and the risk of both tripled. Sadly, these findings held, irrespective of the food choices made (Pereira, 2005).

Since this book is about cancer prevention, we need to ask if there is any indication that a fast food diet can contribute to cancer risk. As discussed earlier, both obesity and diabetes are risk factors for developing cancer and significant increases in both are seen in people who eat fast food fare. The five-to-nine-a-day rule that cuts cancer risk in half would be difficult to achieve by eating fast food alone. Fast food is high in sodium, and a strong association has been shown between high salt intake and gastric cancer. Exposure to acrylamide is a significant concern as well.

In 2002, researchers in Sweden discovered that acrylamide forms during the baking or frying of certain foods, especially starchy foods (Tareke, 2002). Acrylamide, which is present in grout and concrete, has been shown to cause cancer in laboratory animals. A long-term study demonstrated that women who consumed large amounts of french fries when they were children had a higher risk of having breast cancer (Michels, 2005). In 2005, the World Health Organization labeled acrylamide as "probably carcinogenic to humans" and warned that people eat less food containing acrylamide. At the time of this writing, California's attorney general Bill Lockyer has filed suit against nine manufacturers of potato chips and french fries, seeking a court order that consumers be warned that some of their products contain acrylamide. It is estimated that consumers of french fries take in up to 125 times the amount of acrylamide that requires a warning under current regulations. A summary of acrylamide content in certain foods is listed below. Those who are interested in a more detailed list of acrylamide content in foods can find information at www.oehha.ca.gov/prop65/acrylamideintakefdaappendix.pdf.

Table 8-1. Summary of Acrylamide Intake Estimates (OEHHA)

Summary of Acrylamide Intake Estimates (OEHHA)		
Food	**Mean AA (ppb)**	**Intake Range[1] (µg/day)**
Almonds (fried or roasted)	320	0.05 – 0.93
Bagels, untoasted	31	0.28 – 0.43
Biscuits	37	0.15 – 2.37
Bread (soft breads, all types)	**31**	**1.00 – 1.69**
white bread	11	0.29 – 0.77
wheat bread and whole grain	39	0.43 – 2.38
Cake	10	0.09 – 1.00
Cereal, Ready-to-Eat (all types)	**86**	**1.99 – 4.88**
corn flakes[2]	**61**	**1.41 – 3.46**
crisped rice[2]	**56**	**1.29 – 3.18**
granola[2]	**51**	**1.18 – 2.89**
oat rings[2]	**174**	**4.02 – 9.87**
Cereal, cooked, oatmeal, grits, Cream of Wheat	0	0.00 – 0.00
Cereal, cooked, Wheatena	738	?[3] - 30.3
Chicken nuggets/breaded chicken	24	0.21 - ?[3]
Chile con Carne	**130**	**1.05 - ?[3]**
Coffee (brewed)	**7**	**1.71 – 3.73**
Cookies (all types)	**188**	**2.37 – 7.76**
sugar cookies[4]	41	0.52 – 1.69

Summary of Acrylamide Intake Estimates (OEHHA)		
Food	**Mean AA (ppb)**	**Intake Range[1] (µg/day)**
graham cracker[4]	**459**	**5.78 – 19.0**
chocolate chip cookies[4]	**130**	**1.64 – 5.40**
Corn Chips / Tortilla Chips	199	0.80 – 9.15
Crackers	167	0.63 – 3.17
Doughnuts	18	0.07 - 0.85
French fries	**413**	**5.00 – 26.3**
Olives, canned	414	0.28 – 4.14
Pancakes and Waffles	15	0.08 – 1.29
Peanuts, roasted	27	0.04 – 0.55
Peanut butter	88	0.31 – 2.99
Pie	22	0.15 – 3.56
Pizza	20	0.38 – 3.50
Popcorn	180	0.47 – 4.32
Potato Chips	**466**	**2.47 – 14.4**
Postum (dry)	4573	0.01 – 13.7
Prune juice	159	0.09 – 16.4
Quickbreads and muffins	8	0.05 – 0.70
Sunflower seeds	39.5	0.01 – 1.15
Sweet potatoes, canned	84	0.06 – 26.0
Toast	**213**	**1.64 – 7.31**
Tortillas (corn or flour)	6	0.04 – 0.41

Bold type indicates foods whose range of average daily intake exceeds 1.0 µg/day.

1. Intake range is the mean *per capita* intake (lower bound) to the mean intake if one ate the food every day (upper bound). The source of the food consumption data was the CSFII 94-96, 98 survey where possible; otherwise, intake rates based on CSFII 94-96 (Smiciklas et al., 2002) were used. For Wheatena, one serving size as appears on the box label was used as the intake rate.
2. Intake estimates for cereal subtypes assume a person eats that type of cereal solely.
3. Intake data are unavailable.
4. Intake estimates for cookie subtypes assume a person eats that type of cookie solely.

Source: FDA Data on Acrylamide Concentration in Foods. U.S. FDA 2004.
Available at www.oehha.ca.gov/prop65/acrylamideintakefdaappendix.pdf.

Is it possible to eat foods that are somewhat healthy at fast food establishments? In general, foods available on the fast food list include low-quality carbohydrates and foods with a lot of salt and fat, and menus lack fruits and vegetables. Most fast food meals are loaded with 1000 calories, and a single meal may provide a person with a whole day's worth of calories. A single super size-soda alone may provide half of the calories recommended for a day. Trans fat content (which is linked to heart disease and cancer) is also high, with an average medium french fries order having eight grams. Trans fats are discussed later on, but the recommended maximum daily intake is two grams. If you eat at fast food establishments, we offer a few recommendations for eating healthier:

- Switch to salad (but minimize the dressing, which often has as much fat as a burger).
- Order water or iced tea instead of soda.
- Skip the french fries.
- Order burgers with as many vegetables as possible.

We also recommend reading the nutrition information available when you make your choices. A few Web sites list nutritional information about items from the most popular fast food establishments. The Fast Food Nutrition Fact Explorer (www.fatcalories.com/) lists nutritional information from twelve fast food restaurants. Another site, Nutrition Data (www.nutritiondata.com), gives a grade as well as graphic descriptions of the nutritional content of products offered at thirty-five common fast food establishments.

Ideally, learn to be creative with alternatives to fast food. You don't need a free schedule and several hours of preparation time to eat healthy, just a small dose of planning ahead. Preparing meals ahead of time can stop the whining as well as the growling stomachs, without requiring that you expend energy that has long since been drained during the day. There are several books available about meals that can be made ahead of time and frozen. The book *Once a Month Cooking,* by Mary Beth Lagerberg and Mimi Wilson, is an excellent example, and one of the authors has used this as a launch pad, adapting the menu to fit her family's tastes and cancer prevention efforts, with excellent results! Visiting businesses such as

Mix It Up Meals (www.mixitupmeals.com), where you can go and spend a few hours preparing meals to freeze for the month, can decrease the need for last minute, prepackaged or fast foods. Options such as Seattle Sutton (www.seattlesutton.com) are available as well.

To satisfy children who demand fast food in the car, keep some healthy dried fruits and trail mix on hand, with ingredients they like to tide them over. If children are so hungry they need fast food, but not hungry enough to eat something they ordinarily like, say no. If you struggle with saying no to your child, remind yourself that the patterns of eating they are learning in childhood will likely stay with them for a lifetime. Likewise, most overweight children will become overweight adults. An excellent series of books titled *Parenting with Love and Logic*, by Foster Cline M.D. and Jim Fay, provides practical advice about dealing with parenting issues such as these in ways that are refreshing and fun for parents.

A FEW TIPS FOR HEALTHY EATING WITH CHILDREN

- Eat healthy foods yourself: your children are watching.
- Remember, you are the boss and should make the decisions about what foods are in your home.
- Teach your children how to read food labels.
- Eat meals together as a family; turn off the television and ignore the phone.
- If you do not want your kids to eat it, do not buy it.
- Have children help plan a week's worth of meals.
- Do not make children clean their plates.
- When introducing new foods, require that they taste them, but not that they eat an entire portion.
- If playtime interferes with meals, invite your children's friends to join you.

Organically Grown Foods and Ingredients

"Industrialized, chemical-intensive agriculture and our globalized system of distributing food and fiber are literally destroying the earth, driving two billion farmers off the land, and producing a product which is increasingly contaminated. That is why the wave of the future is organic and sustainable, not GMO."

—Ronnie Cummins, Organic Consumers Association

Sales of organic products in the United States rose from 78 million to 6 billion between 1980 and 2006. This trend is expected to continue at a rate of 20 percent per year. In our coupon-cutting, sale-seeking society, what is driving this force to purchase organic foods and products that are frequently more costly? The usual reasons cited are the avoidance of pesticides and environmental concerns, but choosing organic products has implications for health beyond eliminating pesticide residues and risky hormones.

Conventional studies comparing organic to non-organic produce have compared the basic nutrients: proteins, carbohydrates, fats, and vitamin and mineral content. Most of these studies show little difference between the two groups, except with respect to ascorbic acid content, which is higher in organic foods, and nitrates, which are present more often in non-organic foods. Very few studies have been done, however, comparing other elements of food in these two categories, such as the cancer fighting phytochemicals.

Taking into account the fact that the basic nutrients in foods are similar whether organic or non-organic, why would other constituents such as the antioxidant content differ? One explanation is that secondary plant metabolites, such as phenolics, are constituents of vegetables and fruits that function as their "immune system." Plants produce phytochemicals (plant chemicals) such as phenolics to fight off insects and microorganisms. One study examining this concept showed a significantly higher level of phenolics in fruits grown organically (Asami, 2003). It appears that by "protecting" plants from invasion by insects and bacteria with pesticides, we are actually decreasing their need to manufacture cancer-fighting antioxidants!

An interesting study was done at the Danish Institute of Agricultural Sciences comparing the health of rats fed organic foods to that of rats fed conventionally grown foods. Interestingly, the pesticide levels in the food were below detectable limits in both groups. The findings revealed that the rats fed organic foods were healthier, less obese, slept better and had healthier immune systems (Lauridsen, 2005). The benefits of choosing organic foods goes beyond avoiding pesticide residues, it seems.

The information above does not reduce the concern over pesticide exposure, especially with respect to our children. This is reason enough to head to the health food store or organic section of the grocery store. As discussed in the chapter on environment, exposure to pesticides has been clearly documented to increase cancer and doubles the risk of developing leukemia in children. Consuming organic produce does reduce your exposure to pesticides, which can remain even after thorough washings. Children are more vulnerable than adults are to pesticide exposure, since their bodies are undergoing many more changes. The Consumers Union and the Environmental Working Group have studies showing that children are overexposed to pesticides even if the exposure is within legal limits. Some foods are much more likely than others to contain pesticide residues and this will be discussed further below.

In Chapter Six we discussed how we were perplexed about the fact that many countries have a higher life expectancy than that of the U.S., even though their smoking rate is higher than ours. We know that smoking causes cancer and does not enter into the debate, so we presented a few theories to explain this: exercise, obesity, and vacation time. Another variable could be the food we consume. In the United States we rank far below these "higher-life-expectancy countries" in terms of organic farming (see Table 8-1). Interestingly, we found in our travels that the fruits and vegetables we purchased in Austria were less expensive than the produce we purchase in the United States.

Table 8-1. Organic Farming by Country

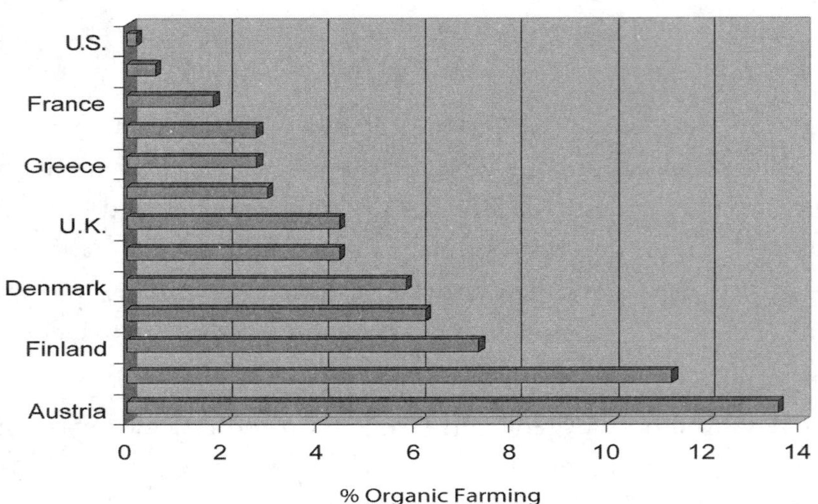

Terms such as "natural" are not regulated and do not indicate that the ingredients are organic. There are specific requirements that need to be met in order for foods to be labeled organic. Some of these requirements are as follows:

- The foods are grown without the use of most conventional pesticides, although some pesticides are allowed.
- No petroleum-based fertilizers are used.
- No sewage sludge-based fertilizers are used.
- No bioengineering has been done (genetically modified food).
- No antibiotics are used.
- No hormones are introduced.

What is the definition of organic? In the United States, products labeled organic must meet the requirements of the Organic Food Production Act of 1990 and the regulations put forth by the USDA through the National Organic Program (NOP). When reading labels the following definitions have been established:

- "100-percent organic" products must be comprised of 100 percent organic ingredients.

- "Organic" products must be made of 95 percent organic ingredients.
- "Made with organic ingredients" describes foods that have 75-90 percent organic ingredients.

Organic produce may not look as appealing as traditionally grown produce, since artificial means (dyes and waxes) are not used to enhance appearance, and in size many organic products are smaller. Many people believe, however, that organic foods taste better. From a consumer standpoint, when you pay more and the food tastes better, you will waste less of it. Look at statistics indicating how much produce goes to waste in our refrigerators; this alone may help justify some of the cost.

So, what organic foods should we purchase? Researchers at the Environmental Working Group (EWG) have selected a list of organically grown fruits and vegetables that they recommend should always be purchased over traditionally grown produce, because of the high pesticide residue on their non-organic equivalents. These include apples, bell peppers, celery, cherries, imported grapes, nectarines, peaches, pears, potatoes, red raspberries, spinach, and strawberries. Keep in mind that this list is based on pesticide residue and does not look at other benefits of organic food.

Those interested in delving deeper into organically grown foods within a budget should see the *Consumer Report Magazine*'s excellent interactive Web site, which discusses when to purchase organically grown foods. This site has a section on testing your organic IQ, and gives you the opportunity to check many products, from produce to meat and dairy, to cosmetics. It provides recommendations that consumers buy organic if possible, buy organic only if cost is not an option, or not to bother buying organic. It can be accessed at www.consumerreports.org/cro/food/organic-products-206/when-buying-organic-pays-and-doesnt.htm. It can also be very helpful to find a good health food store or co-op and get to know the people who work there. Many of these people have a passion for health backed up by a wealth of knowledge they can share to help you make educated food and product choices.

Beef

If you would not normally take hormones and do not need antibiotics, why allow them in your food and hence in you? In the United States, the majority of beef cattle are treated with hormones. It is for this reason that, in 1989, the European Economic Community (EEC) placed a ban on importation of U.S. beef. This ban is still in place. Five hormones are currently used to enhance weight gain in cattle. Three of these are naturally occurring hormones (estrogen, progesterone, and testosterone) and two are synthetic (trenbolene acetate and zeranol). The only approved method of administering hormones to cattle is through implants placed in the cows' ears, although there is concern among some groups that unlawful administration into other sites, such as muscle, could result in much higher concentrations of hormone. Regulations state that residues of hormones in beef must be under one percent of children's daily hormone production. This is very difficult to regulate considering the small number of cattle tested.

Those who support the use of hormones argue that, without administering hormones to stimulate cattle growth and weight gain, ranchers could not afford to produce beef. Hormones generate a 10 to 15 percent increase in weight gain in cattle. We wonder how Europeans afford to buy and produce beef if this is the case. In an era in which the use of estrogen replacement therapy in women has plunged due to studies indicating an increased risk of developing breast cancer, it is concerning that our children consume estrogen in their food.

Fortunately, health food stores, co-ops, and, increasingly, general grocery stores are carrying hormone-free beef products. Make sure to check labels or consult the butcher to make sure the product is indeed hormone free. A label indicating that nothing artificial has been added simply means no artificial ingredients have been added after the animal has been slaughtered. Since many studies talk about an elevated cancer risk with increased consumption of beef, it seems wise to spend a little more money for a purer product, and to eat it less frequently. An Italian study demonstrated an increased risk of developing cancers of the colon, rectum, stomach, pancreas, uterus, ovaries, and breast, in people that ate more than seven servings of red meat per week (Tavani, 2000). Alternatively, try switching to buffalo meat, as a red meat substitute. Buffalo are not usually treated with hormones and antibiotics and buffalo meat is lower in fat than beef by as much as 70-90 percent. An interesting aside: buffalo rarely get cancer, in comparison to other animals! Of note as well is that undercooked buffalo does not pose the danger of spreading E. coli that beef does.

Since buffalo meat is very lean, it should be prepared differently than beef, with shorter cooking times so that it does not become overly dry. If you have not prepared buffalo before, consult your local health food store or one of the buffalo growers associations for recommendations.

Chicken

As we discussed in the last section on beef, we strongly recommend any meat product be hormone free. The health issue related to production of dietary meat, however, goes beyond whether or not the animal has been treated with hormones. If you have had the opportunity to peruse a health food store or the organic section of a grocery store, you may have noted the recent marketing approach heralding "free-range" chicken. Perhaps you are a veteran organic buyer and have already switched to this product.

The advantage of consuming meat from an animal that is free to roam and eat its natural diet, rather than spend its life in a cage eating grains, seems rather obvious. Researchers are now beginning to isolate some of the chemicals that support this. Conjugated linoleic acid (CLA), a powerful cancer-fighting fat, has been found to be most abundant in grass-fed animals. Studies have demonstrated a link between diets high in CLA and a lower risk of developing cancer. Unfortunately, the definition of "free range" is difficult to regulate and only means the chickens are free to go outside for a portion of the day. Likewise, the term "all-natural" is relatively meaningless, meaning only that nothing artificial has been added to the animal product after slaughter. When purchasing chicken, look for labeling that states that the meat is 100 percent organic.

Organic chickens have not been fed growth hormones, antibiotics, or have not been kept tightly in cages. Nor have they been given non-organic feed. Non-organic feed can be laced with toxins and can contain products such as ground-up animal parts, which could, in theory, contribute to contracting mad cow disease. Part of the significantly increased demand for organic dairy products in the recent past has stemmed from this fear, since conventional dairy cows are fed ground-up animal material.

Dairy/BST-Treated milk

Bovine somatotropin (BST), also known as bovine growth hormone (BGH), is a hormone given to dairy cows to increase milk production. The FDA authorized that milk from cows treated with BST be sold unlabeled in 1993, after studies showed milk from BST cows showed no significant differences from that derived from untreated cows. Considerable controversy has been generated worldwide over the safety of this practice. The use of BST has been banned in Australia, New Zealand, and Japan, and was never approved in the European Union countries or in Canada.

BST exerts its effect by acting on insulin-like growth factor (IGF-1), which stimulates growth and, subsequently, milk production in cows. IGF-1, which is structurally identical in cows and humans, is produced naturally in both and regulates cell growth, stimulating growth of both normal and cancerous cells. Concern has been raised that, because natural human IGF-1 has been identified as a growth regulator that accelerates the growth of some types of cancers, theoretically residual IGF-1 in milk from BST-treated cows could increase a consumer's cancer risk. High blood levels of **naturally** occurring IGF-1 have been associated with a significantly increased risk of developing breast, prostate, and colon cancers.

Elevated levels of IGF-1 are found in milk derived from cows treated with BST, but it was thought that the digestive process would break this down, since IGF-1 is a protein. A study published in *JAMA* showed that levels of IGF-1 in this milk are no different from that found in human breast milk, but again this is difficult to interpret, since most adults do not drink human breast milk. Credible sources such as *JAMA* and *Consumer Reports* have published reports reassuring us that milk from BST-treated cows is safe, although questions are still asked in countries where it is banned or not used.

How do we make an informed decision about whether or not to purchase this milk? The authors use a simple, non-scientific approach. It is hard to believe that making a cow produce by artificial means more milk than it is designed to produce is a healthy practice and provides the same product. If there were a shortage of milk in our nation, perhaps this could be justified, but there isn't. Increasing production by using hormones probably helps lower the cost of dairy products for consumers, although the purchase of milk does not deplete most people's checkbooks, and in countries where the use of hormones is banned people still drink milk. The bottom line? Drink hormone-free milk if you can afford it.

Issues regarding the use of BST in cows go beyond a discussion of IGF-1. Cows treated with BST develop mastitis (an udder infection) more frequently, requiring the use of antibiotics. In theory, this would raise our exposure to antibiotics through residual antibiotics in milk, although cows are usually not used for milk production until their infections have cleared. Mastitis in cows is, in fact, the reason that Germany does not allow dairy cows to be treated with BST. In their code of ethics, German veterinarians agree not to intentionally do anything that could inflict harm on animals. Since the use of BST makes cows ill, they deemed its use in dairy cows unethical.

Table 8-2. Foods to Purchase Only if Grown Organically, or if Containing Organically Grown Ingredients

Vegetables:	Fruits:
Bell peppers	Apples
Celery	Cherries
Potatoes	Grapes
Lettuce	Nectarines
Spinach	Peaches
Green beans	Pears
Winter squash	Red raspberries
	Strawberries
Beef (all)	
Chicken (all)	
Dairy: all milk products should have "cows not treated with BST" on the label	
Baby food (all)	

Preparing and Storing Food

"If the divine creator has taken pains to give us delicious and exquisite things to eat, the least we can do is prepare them well and serve them with ceremony."

—Fernand Point

The processes we use to prepare our foods can be as important as the foods themselves. Heating foods can change the nature of the ingredients for better or for worse. Items can be added or formed in the preparation process, as when grilling or using nonstick cookware or plastics. Microbes can grow on stale foods, releasing toxic carcinogens. If we invest the money to purchase a wide variety of healthful organic foods, we should make sure we invest the time to preserve the nutrients without adding contaminants.

Shopping

As discussed above, choosing foods grown organically should be our first priority, but doing so is not always possible or affordable. When selecting produce, try to make choices based on fruits and vegetables that are in season. Some fruits, such as bananas, must be imported given our climate. Practice caution when purchasing imported produce, with an understanding that some imported produce is actually lower in pesticide residues than that grown in the United States.

Cleaning and preparing produce

To get the most of your daily five to nine servings of fruits and vegetables, we offer a few suggestions for preparation:

- Wash all produce, organic and non-organic, thoroughly under running water.
- Peel all fruits and vegetables that are not organic.
- Discard the outer pieces of heads of lettuce.
- Use a brush to scrub potatoes.
- Wash foods even if you are planning on peeling them or cutting them to avoid introducing chemicals and bacteria into the flesh.
- Wax on foods such as apples does not come off with plain water. If you do not peel these fruits, make sure to wash them thoroughly with a safe detergent, such as the commercially available fruit and vegetable washes, and scrub them with a brush.
- Discard the top and bottom one-half inch of bananas before eating.

Ideally, wait to wash and cut produce until just before eating. Washing produce ahead of time can decrease vitamin content, since certain vitamins (vitamin C, folic acid) dissolve in water. In addition, the process of cutting releases an enzyme that begins to destroy vitamin C. We do recommend an exception this general rule, however, and endorse having fresh, cut-up vegetables on hand in the refrigerator. Just as the fast food industry has won over a large segment of the population due to convenience, we will be more likely to eat produce if it is ready in a flash.

In general, eating produce in its most natural state preserves the nutrients and vitamins, and is the healthiest choice. Some exceptions do exist. Steaming broccoli releases more sulphoraphane, the antioxidant that gives broccoli its reputation for helping in preventing cancer. Cooking carrots also increases the antioxidant content, especially if they are left chilled after cooking for a day or two. Steaming is the ideal method of cooking vegetables and it preserves nutrients much better than does boiling or microwaving.

GRILLING

The thought of grilling brings visions of summer picnics and relaxing with friends. Several issues related to grilling and cancer risk have recently surfaced and deserve careful review. When meat is grilled or fried, heterocyclic amines and benzo(a)pyrene, both carcinogens, form on the surface of the meat. Researchers at the University of Minnesota showed that avoiding grilled or fried red meat that is very well done, burned, or charred may help decrease the risk of developing pancreatic cancer (Anderson, 2005). Rather than suggesting that you cancel the picnic, pull out the hose, and douse the grill, we do have suggestions for those that enjoy the taste of grilled foods and want to keep the vision and flavor alive. Many of these ideas take less time than sending the invitations.

- Marinating—Studies have shown that marinating meats prior to grilling reduced the concentration of heterocyclic amines 92 to 99%. This does not have to involve days of preparation. Meats marinated for only 40 minutes showed the same reductions as meats that were marinated for two days. Oil is not a necessary ingredient in marinades and leaving it out can avoid smoking on the grill.
- Meat preparation—Trim away any excess fat before grilling to avoid flare-ups. Avoid using oil in marinades that could drip on the coals and ignite. Consider microwaving meats prior to cooking as well.

Meats that were microwaved for two minutes prior to cooking had a 90% decrease in heterocyclic amine content. Pour off any juices produced when microwaving prior to cooking. Bacon that is microwaved rather than fried is also much lower in heterocyclic amine content.

- Grilling technique – Avoid letting flames touch the meat during cooking. Consider wrapping meat in foil. Shorten the cooking time. A study done by researchers at the National Cancer Institute (NCI) found that people who ate their beef medium well or well done had three times the risk of stomach cancer as those who ate beef rare or medium rare (Ward, 1997). Keep in mind that this applies to cuts of meat such as steak where the inside is not exposed to bacteria. Hamburger should always be cooked thoroughly to avoid infection with a dangerous type of bacteria, *E.coli* 0157:147. Infection with the *E. coli* strain 0157:147 can cause hemorrhagic colitis, hemolytic uremic syndrome (HUS), and Thrombotic thrombocytopenic purpura (TTP), which can be life threatening.
- Prior to serving – Cut away parts of meat that are burned or charred

We also recommend avoiding the use of charcoal lighter fluids. Charcoal lighter fluid contains petroleum distillates that are known carcinogens. Alternatives to lighter fluid include electric starters and fire chimneys. A fire chimney is a round cylinder that can be purchased at barbeque specialty stores and many hardware stores, or even simply made by removing the top and bottom of a metal coffee can. Paper is placed at the bottom with the coals on top. As noted in our discussion of wood burning stoves and fireplaces, make sure to use paper that does not contain dyes or plastic products. If you use lighter fluid, make sure to wait at least forty-five minutes before grilling food. After this amount of time, many of the petroleum byproducts will have dissipated.

Other cooking methods

In general, choose roasting, baking, or boiling over frying, broiling, and grilling. Cooking meats at high temperatures causes the formation of heterocyclic amines. Baking, roasting, and boiling cooks meats at lower temperatures than broiling, frying, and grilling.

Serving temperature of food

Allow foods and beverages to cool slightly prior to serving. The consumption of very high temperature foods and liquids is associated with cancer of the esophagus.

Plastics

Avoid heating plastic and plastic wrap in the microwave; chemicals could leach into the food. Make sure items such as lunchmeats are wrapped in butcher paper at the deli instead of blister packs.

Cooking oil

When cooking with oil, as when sautéing, frying, or deep-frying, discard the used oil and do not reuse it. Every time oil is heated and reheated, more free radicals are produced. Restaurants frequently reheat the oil they use to deep-fry or "top off" the old oil rather than start with fresh. For this reason, as well as for several others, it is best to avoid any deep-fried foods when eating out.

When choosing oils, opt for those containing more omega-3 than omega-6 fatty acids. Animal studies have found that omega-3 fatty acids suppress cancer formation. An increased ratio of omega-3 to omega-6 fatty acids was also found to slow the progression of prostate cancer in mice (Kobayashi, 2006). Omega-3 fatty acids are found in virgin olive oil, flax seed oil, pumpkin seed oil, canola oil, walnut oil, and **non**-hydrogenated soybean oils. Recently, products have shown up on the shelves containing a combination of olive oil and canola oil, which lends itself well to general cooking while having the benefits of the monounsaturated olive oil. Those on a budget might consider making their own combination using any of the above, but make sure to label it.

Cooking pans

We recommend using glass, stainless steel, or ceramic-coated pans for the majority of your cooking. If you would not eat the lining of the pan you are cooking in, do not use it! Perfluoroctanoic acid (PFOA), a chemical used to make Teflon coating, was reported to be a likely human carcinogen by an Environmental Protection Agency advisory panel. PFOA is now found in the blood of 95 percent of Americans. Ideally, it is best to avoid using any pans with a convenient "non-stick" surface. If you do choose to purchase products with a non-stick coating, we recommend you buy upper-end products from well-known manufacturers. Cook at reasonably low temperatures, and discard the pans if they become scratched or if the coating is coming off. Coating the surface of a pan with olive oil can help minimize sticking. To avoid aerosol cans and the fats in less desirable oils and butter, the authors use non-aerosol pumps, which they fill themselves with quality olive oil. If you do choose this method, remember not to spray oil on any heated surface.

Unfortunately, careful selection of cookware alone is not sufficient to avoid all PFOA exposure. Some microwave popcorn bags are treated with a chemical that breaks down to form PFOA and may account for up to 20 percent of the average individual's exposure.

Storing Food/Aflatoxins

Aflatoxins are toxic metabolites produced by fungi in stale foods that can cause liver cancer in humans. Grains and nuts are most often affected, and the highest-risk foods are contaminated and stale corn, peanuts, and cottonseeds. To reduce your chances of ingesting aflatoxins, refrigerate nuts and peanut butter. Store grains in a cool, dark place and toss them if they become stale. The toxin is heat stable, so cooking does not eliminate it. The old adage "if in doubt throw it out" is a good rule to follow with these products.

SUPER-FOODS: HOW TO GET MORE ANTIOXIDANTS FOR YOUR MONEY

"Tomatoes and oregano make it Italian, wine and tarragon make it French. Sour cream makes it Russian, lemon and cinnamon make it Greek. Soy sauce makes it Chinese, garlic makes it good."

—Alice May Brock

One food or dietary plan does not prevent cancer on its own. Consuming a wide variety of foods should be the central theme of a healthy diet. Combining foods provides greater opportunity to ingest substances that may work together to prevent cancer, as shown in a study involving rats. When these rodents consumed broccoli and tomatoes together, the growth rate of tumors was slower than when they ate the vegetables individually in the same amounts (Canene-Adams, 2005). It is, therefore, with hesitation that we present some of the foods that stand out as winners in cancer prevention research and begin this discussion with a dietary approach rather than an endorsement of a single food.

THE MEDITERRANEAN DIET

Many studies have demonstrated a decreased risk of developing cancer with consumption of a Mediterranean diet and, according to a study in *The New England Journal of Medicine* in 2003, this diet is associated with a reduction in death from **all** causes (Trichopoulou, 2003). Several studies have looked at the individual foods and nutrients found in this diet, but the benefit of the overall Mediterranean diet seems to go beyond the benefits measured from individual foods. Perhaps dietary patterns and the combination of foods are the key factors. Components of a typical Mediterranean diet include:

- an emphasis on non-hydrogenated plant oils, particularly the liberal use of olive oil
- breads, potatoes, and grains (unrefined cereals, pasta, couscous, rice, polenta, bulgar)

- fish ranking ahead of red meat, poultry, and eggs
- a multitude of fruits and vegetables
- legumes (chick peas, lentils, beans, peas and peanuts)
- tree nuts (almonds, pistachios, walnuts and hazelnuts)
- seeds (sesame seeds)

Many excellent Mediterranean cookbooks that incorporate these foods into recipes are available. Most children would be pleased that, within the context of a typical Mediterranean diet, the regular consumption of pizza was correlated with a decreased risk of developing digestive tract cancers!

Green Tea

Drinking tea for health is a 5000-year-old tradition in China and India that is now catching on in America with exuberance, as scientists discover concrete evidence supporting this time-honored practice. Many studies have demonstrated a protective effect of green tea against the development of cancers, especially those of the stomach, esophagus, breast, and bladder (Nakachi, 2003; Sun, 2002; Wu, 2003; Zeegers, 2001). Smokers who drink green tea have decreased oxidative DNA damage, which is the set-up for cancer (Hakim, 2004). Interestingly, in Asia, where much of the world's green tea is consumed, there is a significantly lower rate of lung cancer despite a rate of smoking higher than that in the United States..

Many studies using cell cultures and animals show that consuming green tea and the antioxidants found in green tea, catechins, decreases the size and number of tumors and may inhibit the growth of cancer cells (Fujimoto, 2002; Baliga, 2005). Human studies have also shown promise that green tea may have a treatment role in those already diagnosed with cancer. Green tea may prevent breast cancer reoccurrence (Inoue, 2001), and enhance survival in those diagnosed with ovarian cancer (Zhang, 2004). Interestingly, following the unexpected regression of cancer in a few patients who self-initiated treatment with green tea, a National Cancer Institute-sponsored trial of de-caffeinated green tea extracts for patients with early stage chronic lymphocytic leukemia was begun at the Mayo Clinic in 2005 (Shanafelt, 2006).

While black tea may have some protective effect, it is much more processed than is green tea or white tea, as the tea leaves are allowed to ferment and oxidize, thereby developing their darker color. Based on studies reviewed, the authors "practice what they preach" and recommend drinking two to four cups of green tea daily. Green tea should be enjoyed without milk or cream, which possibly inactivates the catechins in tea, and the tea should be steeped for at least five minutes to release the majority of antioxidants. This is a lot of tea, so if you choose to drink decaffeinated green tea, choose one that is decaffeinated by natural means, and purchase organic tea when possible. Drinking green tea also lowers cholesterol, blood pressure, and helps prevent strokes.

Water

A study demonstrated that Taiwanese men who consumed the most water had a 92% lower risk of colorectal cancer than men who drank the least amount (Tang, 1999). A high water intake has also been correlated with a decreased risk of bladder cancer, and in at least one study the risk of breast cancer was decreased by a diet including a high water intake. A diet high in water would conceptually lead to a reduction in cancer for a few reasons. It has been shown that drinking eight glasses per day of water helps with weight control and as stated previously, being overweight is the second leading preventable cause of cancer. High water intake also decreases transit time through the bowel and urinary system and should result in less exposure time to possible carcinogens as well.

Cruciferous vegetables

The majority of studies conducted to date show an inverse association between intake of cruciferous vegetables (such as broccoli and cauliflower) and cancer risk, especially for cancers of the lung and digestive tract. Cruciferous vegetables are high in glucosinolate content. The activity of glucosinolate in the body may help eliminate carcinogens and prevent normal cells from becoming cancerous. Other vegetables classified as cruciferous include: cabbage, brussel sprouts, Chinese cabbage, bok choy, mustard greens, kale, collard greens, kohlrabi, kale, turnips, rutabaga, arugula, wasabi, radishes, and horseradish.

Tomato products

Many large studies have documented a significant reduction in the incidence of prostate cancer in men who consume foods rich in lycopene. Lycopene also appears to protect against heart disease and has anti-inflammatory properties. Lycopene is a compound found in high amounts in tomatoes, and is also found in watermelon. When tomatoes are crushed and cooked, more lycopene is released than in raw tomatoes and therefore tomato sauces are an ideal food choice. It is noteworthy that the incidence of prostate cancer is much lower in southern Mediterranean countries where tomato sauces are celebrated.

Blueberries

Blueberries are rich in anthrocyanosides, which are currently the second most powerful antioxidants known to researchers.

Fish

Fish are high in omega-3 fatty acids, which, along with selenium, are being studied for their role in cancer prevention. In one study, prostate cancer was two to three times more common in men who ate no fish than it was in men who ate moderate to large amounts of fish (Terry, 2001). Although study results are mixed, fish consumption may play a protective role against the development of several other cancers as well. If you are not a big fish lover, it is encouraging that data from a series of studies in Italy showed that consumption of even relatively small amounts of fish decreased the risk of several cancers (Fernandez, 1999). Cold-water, fatty fish such as salmon, tuna, and mackerel are ideal choices.

Mercury content in fish has been increasing in recent years. To minimize exposure consider alternating between different types of fish. Choose "wild" fish over farm-raised fish when available. If you eat lake fish, be aware of recommendations about how frequently you should eat different types of fish, based on the lakes fished. The Environmental Protection Agency hosts a Web site, "Windows to My Environment," where, based on zip code and city, citizens can access information about the lakes where they fish and view recommendations on frequency of fish consumption. This is available at www.epa.gov/enviro//wme/. Pregnant women should avoid certain fish, including salmon, swordfish, mackerel, and snapper, and should follow recommendations regarding lake fish carefully.

FLAX

Flax is rich in omega-3 fatty acids that, in addition to having a protective effect against cancer, are beneficial in the prevention of other diseases as well. Choose breads that contain flax seed or add it to your bread recipes. Flax seed does contain lignans that have a phytoestrogen effect; therefore, women with estrogen receptor-positive tumors may want to discuss whether to eat flax with their physicians.

APPLES—AN ORGANIC APPLE A DAY MAY KEEP THE ONCOLOGIST AWAY

The National Cancer Institute has reported that foods containing flavenoids, like those found in apples, may reduce the risk of lung cancer by up to 50 percent (Marchand, 2000). With lung cancer estimated to claim over 162,000 lives in the U.S. in 2006, an apple a day could save the lives of 80,000 Americans a year. Perhaps if it were not for Johnny Appleseed, the incidence of lung cancer in the U.S. would be higher yet!

What types of apples should you choose? We first recommend any apple you will eat, because eating the poorest quality apple is better than letting the highest quality one rot in the refrigerator. If you do not have a preference, a study in Canada of eight types of apples revealed Red Delicious to have the highest antioxidant content. This study also showed that the skin of the apple contained five times more antioxidants than the flesh, so we strongly recommend purchasing organic apples and eating the skin when palatable (Tsao, 2005). Apple cider is made using whole apples, including the skins, and is preferable over apple juice for this reason. Make sure to purchase organic cider.

Collard greens, spinach, and kale

Collard greens are very high in lutein, which has been associated with a decreased risk of developing breast, lung, and colon cancers. While many vegetables contain lutein, levels are particularly high in collard greens, spinach, kale, and turnip and mustard greens. Lutein also appears to play a protective role against developing cataracts and macular degeneration. Try to eat a food in this category daily. Women who ate at least six servings of spinach, kale, and other green vegetables a week had half the risk of developing ovarian cancer as did women who consumed less than two servings per week (Kushi, 1999).

Olive oil

Countries in which the greatest amount of olive oil is consumed (Greece, Italy) have one-third the incidence of breast cancer that the United States has. In Italy, individuals who consumed the highest amounts of olive oil had a decreased incidence of pancreatic cancer (LeVecchia, 1997). Olive oil is an important component of the Mediterranean diet, which as noted previously, is associated with a lower mortality rate, including that associated with cancer. A heavy pocketbook is not required in order to cook healthy meals with olive oil. We recommend a good quality, general use, organic, extra virgin olive oil.

Kelp/seaweed

Japanese women, who have a much higher dietary intake of seaweed, have a significantly lower risk of breast cancer than do women in the United States. Animal studies suggest that seaweed exerts its effect by lowering estrogen levels, resulting in a lower risk of developing breast cancer. There are additional benefits to eating seaweed. Women who consume greater amounts of kelp have more days between menstrual cycles (less frequent periods) and experience significantly less menstrual pain than do those who eat lesser amounts (Skibola, 2005). In Japan, seaweed is used in sushi, miso soup, stews, as a thickening agent, and as a snack. Seaweed products such as kelp can be purchased at health food stores and are easy to add to soups or eat as a snack. Check out cookbooks or online recipes to find palatable ways of adding seaweed to your diet.

BEANS

Countries with the highest bean consumption have a lower death rate from breast, prostate, and colon cancer. In addition to aiding in prevention, saponins, a phytochemical found in beans, might prevent cancer cells already present from multiplying. Current dietary guidelines published by the USDA recommend three cups of beans per week. Most American diets are well below that recommendation. The response we expect from this: what about the gas? Tips to decrease gas experienced from eating beans include soaking dry beans overnight before cooking, discarding the soaking water, and rinsing the beans. If necessary, use a preparation such as Beano®. Symptoms can also be minimized by increasing the amount of beans in your diet slowly.

RASPBERRIES AND STRAWBERRIES

Strawberries and raspberries are rich in ellagic acid, which may play a role in the prevention of skin, bladder, lung, and breast cancers. Ellagic acid works as an anti-oxidant and has also been shown to slow the reproduction of cancer cells.

RED GRAPES

Red grapes contain resveratrol, which helps to protect a person against cancer in several ways. It has anti-inflammatory properties (as discussed earlier, inflammation can cause cancer), works as an anti-oxidant (neutralizing free radicals), and slows the progression of abnormal cells into cancer. Reservatrol levels are especially high in red grapes and red wine. Caution needs to be exercised, however, and the authors recommend any product containing alcohol for health reasons be limited only to those who are at a very low risk for becoming addicted. A European study demonstrated a decreased risk of developing breast cancer in people eating red grapes but not drinking red wine (Levi, 2005). Although this study didn't give reasons, we know that alcohol intake in women is associated with an increased risk of developing breast cancer. The foil around corks can also contaminate wine with lead (a known carcinogen). If you purchase wine, try to buy organic varieties and bottles without foil around the corks.

Broccoli sprouts

Broccoli sprouts have levels of sulphoraphane, a compound believed to help prevent colon cancer, in amounts much greater than those found in broccoli alone.

Brazil nuts

Brazil nuts are very high in selenium, a mineral that is increasingly becoming known for its cancer-prevention role and discussed further when we address super vitamins and minerals. A one-ounce serving of Brazil nuts (six to eight nuts) contains 543 ug of selenium. The upper intake level recommended daily is 400 ug, so eat just a few on occasion.

Pineapple

Pineapple contains bromelain, a compound shown to decrease cancer in animals.

Pomegranates

Pomegranates are rich in antioxidants. Studies have shown that pomegranate juice helps protect against sun damage from UVA rays (Syed, 2006). Pomegranate extract also appears to play a protective role against the development of prostate cancer, and may slow the growth of prostate, colon and breast cancers (Pantuck, 2006; Adams, 2006; Jeune, 2005; Malik 2005).

Avocados

Avocados are rich in glutathione, a strong antioxidant. Other good sources of glutathione include watermelon, asparagus, potatoes, and grapefruits. Some researchers believe avocados may help treat viral hepatitis as well, which is one cause of liver cancer, as noted previously.

Exotic mushrooms

Mushrooms such as shiitake, maitake, and oyster contain the powerful antioxidant L-ergothionene. In addition to possibly preventing some cancers from developing, they are increasingly being used in alternative remedies for treating cancer.

Sweet potatoes

Sweet potatoes are very high in vitamin C, B-carotene, and folate, which have all been shown to play a protective role against cancer in some studies. Baked or fried sweet potatoes could provide a healthier alternative for those who crave french fries.

Carrots

Animal research has demonstrated a decreased risk of developing cancer with consumption of carrots. In contrast to most foods, which are best eaten in the least processed way possible, when cooked their cancer-fighting potential increases. In a University of Arkansas study, the antioxidant content in carrots increased over 30 percent with cooking and continued to increase for the first week of storage (Talcott, 2000). Until studies show us that the same is true of other vegetables, the rule remains: the freshest and least processed products are best. If you enjoy your time in the sun at the beach, pack some carrot sticks in your beach bag. Carrots can help protect your skin from the solar damage that leads to skin cancer.

Dark chocolate

Dark chocolate contains polyphenols, powerful antioxidants. Milk chocolate contains these as well, but a candy bar of dark chocolate contains as many polyphenols as would be consumed in two days' worth of eating fruits and vegetables. Before becoming a chocoholic, keep in mind that there is more to vegetables than polyphenols, and chocolate can be high in fat and calories.

GRAINS, TUBERS, LEGUMES, AND ROOTS

Whole grains, tubers, legumes, and roots are potential cancer fighters, but only 5 percent of Americans get three servings per day, more or less the recommended seven servings per day. According to the FDA, foods must contain at least 51 percent whole grains, that is, grain with all three of the kernels intact, to be labeled whole grain. To ensure you are buying foods containing whole grains, look at the list of ingredients. For example, buy products that list whole-wheat flour, not enriched wheat flour, on the label. Examples of these foods include:

- Grains – whole wheat flour (also known as graham flour), cracked wheat (bulgur), oatmeal, rolled oats, quick oats, brown rice, whole cornmeal, whole grain barley
- Tubers – sweet potatoes
- Legumes – beans, peas, lentils
- Roots – beets, turnips, parsnips, rutabagas

HOT CHOCOLATE

Hot cocoa has more antioxidants than does red wine (two times) or green tea (three times) and only one-third the fat of a chocolate bar.

GARLIC

High consumption of allium vegetables, such as garlic, is associated with a lower risk of having stomach and colon cancer. Other allium vegetables include chives, onions, leeks, and shallots.

ROSEMARY

Carnosol, an extract of rosemary, inhibits the development of breast and skin cancers in animals.

TUMERIC

Tumeric is a spice rich in antioxidants and is found in items such as curry powder and mustard. In animal studies, tumeric hinders the growth of cancers, including breast, skin and colon cancers, as well as lymphomas. While eating tumeric offers hope as a cancer prevention method, be aware that it can interfere with a few chemotherapy medications and, as stated early on, should only be used by cancer patients under direction of their physicians.

GINGER

Ginger has been shown in studies to decrease the growth of colon cancer cells.

SUPER-FOODS SUMMARY

Fill your pantry and fridge with a healthy variety of these foods. To assist you in compiling your shopping list, the U.S. Department of Agriculture has evaluated many foods extensively, and has provided a ranking of the top twenty food sources of antioxidants. These are listed in Table 8-3.

Table 8-3. Top 20 Sources of Antioxidants

THE U.S. DEPARTMENT OF AGRICULTURE'S RANKING OF THE TOP 20 SOURCES OF ANTIOXIDANTS:

1. Small red beans, dry, ½ cup	11. Strawberries, 1 cup
2. Wild blueberries, 1 cup	12. Red delicious apples, 1
3. Red kidney beans, ½ cup	13. Granny Smith apples, 1
4. Pinto beans, dry, ½ cup	14. Pecans, 1 ounce
5. Cultured blueberries, 1 cup	15. Sweet cherries, 1 cup
6. Cranberries, 1 cup	16. Black plums, 1
7. Artichoke hearts, 1 cup	17. Russet potatoes, cooked, 1
8. Blackberries, 1 cup	18. Black beans, dried, ½ cup
9. Prunes, ½ cup	19. Plums, 1
10. Raspberries, 1 cup	20. Gala apples, 1

Source: Wu, X. et al. 2004. Lipophilic and Hydrophilic Antioxidant Capacities of Common Foods in the United States. *Journal of Agricultural and Food Capacity.* 52:4026-4037.

Super-vitamins, Nutrients, and Foods That Contain Them

"Human beings do not eat nutrients, they eat food."

—Mary Catherine Bateson

As noted in the section on super-foods, we hesitate to isolate specific vitamins that play a role in cancer prevention, since the emphasis of a cancer prevention diet should be on variety. A few vitamins and minerals stand out, however, and incorporating foods containing these into your daily diet may provide added benefits. We list some foods that are good sources of the vitamins discussed, but knowing that the tastes and preferences of different individuals vary considerably, we refer those with an interest to an excellent Web site that lists the nutritional and vitamin content of many foods. On this site, you'll find information about items from vitamin A to selenium to fiber, and you can obtain a list of foods that contain these elements, arranged according to degree of content. You can access the USDA National Nutrient Database at www.ars.usda.gov/Services/docs.htm?docid=9673.

Selenium

Selenium is a mineral that is rapidly developing a reputation for its role in preventing cancer. Many studies show a reduction in several cancer types in people who consume dietary or supplemental selenium. Selenium content in soil varies across the country and has been postulated as one of the factors accounting for geographical differences in the incidence of cancer. Selenium levels in soil are highest in the plains states, especially Nebraska and the Dakotas, and very low in China and Russia. Heavily farmed soil is low in selenium, another reason to purchase organically grown food when possible. Brazil nuts stand out as having the highest amount of selenium by a factor of five, but other good sources include mixed nuts, seafood, and whole grain wheat flour.

Be aware that selenium has a narrow therapeutic window. This means that it is protective, but too much can be toxic. The recommended daily allowance for selenium is 55 ug per day for men and women ages nineteen and older, with a maximum recommended level of 400 ug per day. Most people in the United States, except those with gastrointestinal problems such as Crohn's disease, get the minimum recommendation for selenium in their diets. Toxicity is quite rare but results in a condition called selenosis. Symptoms of selenosis include gastrointestinal upset; hair loss; garlic-scented breath; fatigue; white, patchy nails; and minor neurological symptoms.

Vitamin B6

A healthy intake of vitamin B6 is important, especially for those who consume alcohol. A large study in Sweden showed a 34 percent lower incidence of colon cancer in women who consumed high dietary levels of vitamin B6 compared to those who had low levels. The results were even more dramatic for the women in the study who consumed two or more servings of alcohol per week. In this group, there was a 72 percent lower incidence of colon cancer in women who had high intakes of vitamin B6 (Larsson, 2005). Good dietary sources of vitamin B6 include green leafy vegetables, citrus fruits, dried beans, peas, and fortified cereals.

Folic acid

Inadequate intake of folic acid has been associated with the development of cancer. Folic acid exerts its effect by preventing DNA mutations that can lead to cancer later in life. Folic acid plays a protective role against prostate cancer and may be helpful in fighting early cervical cancer. Studies have been done suggesting that folic acid may reduce the increased risk of developing breast cancer from alcohol consumption, but results have been mixed (Tjonneland, 2006; Stolzenberg-Solomon, 2006). Foods that are high in folic acid include green leafy vegetables, blackberries, raspberries, sunflower seeds, oranges, and tangerines.

The majority of our nutritional recommendations place emphasis on a dietary approach alone. With regard to folic acid, a supplement may be beneficial. The Nurses' Health Study, a large study involving nearly 90,000 women conducted by Harvard, showed that women who took a 400 mcg supplement of folic acid daily for fifteen years had a 75 percent reduction in colon cancer (Giovannucci, 1998). People taking methotrexate to treat cancers and other disorders should not use folic acid.

Vitamin A

Having a diet low in vitamin A may increase your risk of developing cancer. In the above study of 90,000 nurses, those who were in the top 20 percent of vitamin A intake (through diet or the use of supplements) were much less likely to develop breast cancer than those in the lower 20 percent (Hunter, 1993). High levels of vitamin A can be toxic and can cause birth defects in utero. This is probably not a concern with reasonable dietary intake alone. Most supplements contain 10,000 to 25,000 IUs per day and pregnant women should not consume more than 10,000 IUs per day. Smokers should also exhibit caution, since there is some evidence that supplements containing vitamin A and beta-carotene may increase the risk of lung cancer developing in smokers (Omenn, 1996). Good dietary sources of vitamin A include turkey, carrots, pumpkins, sweet potatoes, and spinach.

Vitamin D

Vitamin D has been shown for some time to play a protective role against prostate cancer. Researchers now believe that daily intake of 1000 IU of vitamin D reduces the risk of cancers of the colon, breast, and ovary as well (Garland, 2006). For promoting bone health, current recommendations for vitamin D are 200 IUs daily for people between the ages of one and fifty, 400 IUs daily for those fifty-one to seventy years of age, and 600 IUs daily thereafter. These recommendations may change, as studies show doses of 1000 to 1500 IUs per day may help prevent medical conditions beyond osteoporosis, including cancer (Birschoff-Ferrari, 2006). An 8-ounce glass of milk supplies approximately 100 IUs. Spending ten to fifteen minutes in the sun outdoors on a sunny day with 40 percent of the body exposed can result in the absorption of a major 2000-5000 IUs.

Fiber

Adequate dietary intake of fiber in European studies has shown a protective effect against developing colorectal cancer. A study published in *Lancet* postulated that people with a low average intake of fiber could decrease their risk of developing colon cancer 40 percent by doubling their daily intake of fiber. This study, done in Europe, settled on 35 grams of fiber per day as the effective amount (Bingham,

2003). U.S. studies reviewed by the authors have created controversy recently, as results have demonstrated a lack of a protective effect from fiber in cereals, fruits, and vegetables. These studies used lower amounts of fiber than did the European studies, with a range of 10 to 30 grams per day (Park, 2005).

Interestingly, a diet high in fiber has been shown to decrease the risk of girls having their first menstrual periods early by almost 50 percent, and having later first periods is associated with a lower incidence of breast cancer (Rohan, 2002). High fiber diets could also theoretically decrease the risk of developing breast cancer by decreasing the intestinal reabsorption of estrogen.

The average American takes in only about 11 grams of fiber per day. This is much lower than the National Cancer Institute's recommendation of 20 to 30 grams per day. If you decide to increase your dietary fiber intake, do so slowly! A rapid increase in dietary fiber can cause gas and bloating and subsequently a tendency to give up!

Foods, Vitamins, and Minerals and Controversies About Them

"All I ask of food is that it doesn't harm me."

—Michael Palin, *Monty Python's Flying Circus*

Milk

Studies evaluating the intake of milk and dairy products have yielded mixed results. Based on a review of the literature, it seems that moderation is the key regarding intake. Recent studies have shown that people who consumed at least one glass of milk per day were less likely to get colorectal cancer (Larsson, 2006; Cho, 2004). Studies, however, looking at high intake have shown an association between milk and the development of prostate and ovarian cancer (Gao, 2005; Larsson, 2006). Other factors such as calcium may play a role as well. Several of the studies evaluated were European-based, where BST has been banned, and therefore milk from BST-treated cows is probably not a factor in these results.

Calcium

A recent study did not show any benefit of taking calcium to postmenopausal women with respect to reducing their odds of getting colon cancer (Wactawski-Wende, 2006). Prior to this study, presented in *The New England Journal of Medicine*, calcium had long been considered to play a role in reduction of colon cancer. Patients receiving adequate intake of calcium (1200 grams/day) had been shown to be less likely to experience the regrowth of polpys, one type of which is the precursor to colon cancer (Baron, 1999). Before tossing out the calcium bottle, know that the women in the *New England Journal* study did have an improvement in their hip bone density (Jackson, 2006). This book is focused on cancer prevention, but hip fractures are just as devastating in many ways, causing significant disability and premature death. As with dairy products, an excess intake of calcium may increase the risk of developing prostate cancer in men and moderation is key (Gao, 2005).

Soy

Studies evaluating the role of soy in cancer prevention have also yielded mixed results, some showing benefit and some showing no benefit (Trock, 2006). Soy products have been evaluated for possible cancer prevention properties, based on observations that populations that consume more soy have a lower risk of developing some cancers. While soy may be associated with a small reduction in incidences of breast cancer, some studies with human breast cancer cells show that soy can actually promote tumor growth. We could speculate that the estrogen-like effects of soy are preventative before a tumor starts but accelerate growth once a tumor develops. Or perhaps soy has different effects in premenopausal versus postmenopausal women, but until more is known, we recommend caution. From a prevention standpoint, go ahead and eat tofu and soy nuts if you enjoy them. Though the question about soy's role in cancer remains unanswered, soy is a healthier option as a source of protein than beef.

VITAMIN E

After long being touted for its effectiveness in heart disease and cancer prevention, supplemental vitamin E has been sent to the witness stand for further questioning. Perhaps the form of vitamin E is most important in the controversy. A team of researchers at M.D. Anderson Cancer Center studied two forms of vitamin E. One form, alpha-tocopherol, significantly decreased a person's risk of developing bladder cancer, while another form, gamma-tocopherol, offered no benefit (Hernandez, 2004). Foods high in alpha-tocopherol include almonds, red and green peppers, sunflower seeds, mustard greens, spinach, and vegetable oils.

MULTIVITAMINS

Medical opinions are mixed about taking a daily multivitamin. Studies have given support to those on both sides of the fence without a thundering cry to lean one way or the other (Lichtenstein, 2005). In our unscientific poll of fellow healthcare professionals, we have seen people gather on both sides; some take vitamins and some don't. Both sides are probably correct. A daily multivitamin is probably not necessary if you eat five to nine servings of organically grown fruits and vegetables per day. If you, however, consume the typical American diet of only one fruit and one vegetable daily, you are probably deficient in the basic vitamins and minerals necessary for good immune function. Based on federal recommendations, only 10 percent of adults and 2 percent of children eat a healthy diet (Basiotis, 2002, Munoz, 1997). The addition of a multivitamin is most important for those with poor dietary practices, the elderly, and those with excessive alcohol consumption, where alcohol is replacing nutrients in the diet.

In general, the daily use of a multivitamin is safe. Most vitamins and minerals are water-soluble and excreted when taken in excess. The fat-soluble vitamins A, D, E and K, however, can be stored in the body and build up if taken in excess. This is not usually a concern with a multivitamin, with the exception of vitamin A. An excess of vitamin A can cause birth defects in the fetuses of pregnant women exposed to excessive levels. (See our discussion of vitamin A in the super vitamins section for exposure limits.)

The use of **antioxidant supplements** has also become common since they were released onto the "free" market a decade ago. Studies evaluating the role of antioxidants in cancer prevention have been inconsistent, but a few have demonstrated taking antioxidants to be beneficial in preventing the development of cancer. A study in China involving 30,000 people who took an antioxidant supplement showed the supplement users had a 13 percent decrease in expected cancer deaths over a five year period (Blot, 1994). A recent study in Quebec showed a 48 to 54 percent reduction in prostate cancer in men who took antioxidant vitamins and mineral supplements (Meyer, 2005). In contrast, two large-scale studies demonstrated an **increase** in the development of lung cancer in **smokers** that took antioxidant supplements (Omenn, 1994; The Alpha-Tocopheral, Beta Carotene Cancer Prevention Study Group, 1994).

For now, we recommend that smokers avoid antioxidant supplements especially those containing beta carotene, vitamin A, and vitamin E. If you are a non-smoker and choose to use an antioxidant supplement, ask for advice from your physician or nutrition specialist about how to choose a quality product since available products vary widely in their quality and active ingredients. In addition, as noted previously, if you have been diagnosed with cancer and are undergoing treatment, taking some supplements could interfere with your therapy, and careful discussion with your oncologist is imperative.

COFFEE

If you like to relax with a cup of coffee in the morning...relax! A large study involving 90,000 people in Toyko found that middle-aged and elderly people who drank coffee (most of the subjects drank regular coffee) were only half as likely to develop liver cancer as were non-coffee drinkers (Inoue, 2005). Regular consumption of decaffeinated coffee, but not regular, has been shown to reduce the risk of developing rectal cancer (Michels, 2005). This is not an overwhelming reason to start a new habit but is reassuring to those who like to jumpstart their day with a cup of java. Heavy coffee consumption (more than five cups of coffee daily), however, is sited as a possible cause of bladder cancer (Villanueva, 2006).

If you choose to drink decaffeinated coffee, choose products that are decaffeinated by the Swiss water decaffeination method or by the carbon dioxide method rather than those decaffeinated by chemical solvents. Check the package for the method used. Trichloroethylene, which was once used to decaffeinate coffee, was tested by the National Cancer Institute (NCI) and shown to cause liver tumors in mice. In the 1970s coffee manufacturers began to use other solvents, including methylene chloride, ethyl acetate, and others. Now methylene chloride is strongly suspected to be a carcinogen and is rarely used.

We also recommend coffee lovers use unbleached coffee filters. According to the Environmental Protection Agency (EPA), using bleached coffee filters can result in a lifetime dioxin (a carcinogen) level that exceeds acceptable levels.

Carbonated beverages

The increased consumption of carbonated beverages has been correlated in studies and discussions with the risk of developing adenocarcinoma of the esophagus, a risk that has tripled since the 1970s. Since drinking carbonated beverages increases gastric pressure, which in turn can cause reflux, and reflux is the most important risk factor for this type of cancer, this correlation made sense to many investigators. A recent study examining the link, however, did not show an increase in cancer in drinkers of carbonated beverages and actually showed a decrease in people consuming the most carbonated beverages (Mayne, 2006). Regardless of whether the next study shows that carbonated beverages increase or decrease cancer risk, we know that many of our children are replacing good nutrients with the empty calories in soda. Obesity continues to rise and osteoporosis can be expected to as well, since both can result from drinking too much soda. Best bet: limit the number of soft drinks you consume.

Microwaving foods

With the exception of cooking red meat, where microwaving may decrease exposure to carcinogens, microwave preparation of foods raises some concerns. Microwaving may destroy a significant amount of some vitamins and phytochemicals in food and therefore may frustrate their protective effects against cancer. One study that evaluated the effect of several cooking methods on the antioxidant content of broccoli demonstrated that microwaving destroyed 97 percent of flavenoids. Boiling removed 47 to 66 percent of the flavenoids, while steaming had little effect (Vallejo, 2003). Another study evaluated vitamin B12 in food and found that it was inactivated by microwave heating (Watanobe, 1998). In researching the effects of microwaving on food, the authors found a paucity of information and few scientific studies. This came as a surprise, since 90 percent of homes in the United States include a microwave.

One area that has been more widely publicized is the effect of heating breast milk in the microwave. A study in *Pediatrics* found that the microwaving process destroyed 98 percent of the antibodies present in the milk (Yang, 1992). It is well known that microwaving baby bottles is not recommended since the milk can heat in an irregular fashion and burn babies' mouths, or the bottle can explode due to the build-up of steam. This study implies that the time and energy mothers spend pumping to provide breast milk that will decrease their babies' risk of getting infections may be in vain if the milk is heated in the microwave.

It is clear that other changes in microwaved substances take place as well. In a highly published account in 1991, a woman in Oklahoma was killed by a blood transfusion. Instead of using the conventional method of heating blood prior to transfusion, the blood was heated in a microwave oven. Changes in proteins in the blood subsequently caused a fatal allergic reaction.

The relevance of this to people and other substances and foods is less clear. Conventional heating also changes food substances, and, as noted with meats, may increase a person's exposure to carcinogens. This area needs much further research and evaluation. For now we recommend avoiding heating breast milk in the microwave, and opting for steaming rather than microwaving vegetables.

Low-fat diet

The "low-fat diet" was popularized when the testing of cholesterol became routine and has become the approach for many a health-conscious individual seeking weight loss. Diets high in fat have been associated with cancers of the breast, colon, prostate, and uterus. The typical American consumes approximately 40 percent of calories from fat. An initial goal should be 30 percent or less of daily calories from fat, with an ideal goal of less than 20 percent. Results of the Women's Health Initiative study published in 2006 were disappointing, as the media publicized that a low-fat diet did nothing to reduce the risk of developing breast or colon cancer (Beresford, 2006; Prentice, 2006). Does this mean we can reject earlier studies and confidently return to our 40 percent fat diet without guilt? Analyzing the methodology of studies is important before drawing abrupt conclusions. In this study, women were supposed to cut their fat calories to 20 percent of their daily caloric intake to accurately test the effects of a low-fat diet. In fact, closer to 30 percent of their caloric intake was from fat. Women who started out eating the most fat did have a significantly lower breast cancer risk after lowering fat intake. It could also be that a study done over a longer time period would be required to show a difference. Perhaps the type of fats consumed could be relevant. Possibly, a lack of cancer reduction when we decrease fat in our diets is due to the nutrients we substitute for fats, such as corn syrup and refined sugar. Ironically, despite the introduction of the low-fat version of a multitude of foods, America's waistline continues to widen.

This is also an area where going to either extreme can be dangerous. Some fat is necessary in a healthy diet to absorb the fat-soluble vitamins A, D, E, and K, and very low-fat diets actually increase the risk of developing cancer.

Suggestions to help you decrease the fat in your diet:

- Avoid fried foods. Choose alternatives such as baked, roasted, and boiled.
- Remove skin from chicken and turkey.
- Choose lean cuts of beef.
- Choose buffalo over beef to satisfy cravings for red meat.
- Eat more fish.
- Choose tuna canned in water rather than in oil.
- Choose low-fat dairy products.
- Try herbs and spices instead of butter or margarine for seasoning.
- Substitute olive oil for butter or margarine.

- Consume smaller portions of high-fat food.
- Ask for sauces, salad dressings, and gravy on the side.

Foods and Food Additives to Minimize or Avoid

"We are living in a world today where lemonade is made from artificial flavors and furniture polish is made from real lemons."

—Alfred E. Newman

Except for a poisonous fish in Asia considered a delicacy, and certain mushrooms, very few foods are dangerous on their own. Essentially, this section addresses innovations to improve the aesthetics, taste, and shelf-life of foods. Some of these practices, such as smoking and curing foods, were necessary in years past to avoid more immediately threatening problems such as malnutrition or illness from eating rancid food. Some are more recent practices aimed at preserving our food. These allow us to live our lives more spontaneously, shopping when we wish to and knowing the food will last. Unlike the simple additives listed in the past, complex-sounding ingredients are listed on many food labels. Physicians are warned about potential drug interactions, which increase dramatically with the number of medications a patient takes. We should be cautious of these chemicals that are added to our food but are not naturally existing compounds in food. If you cannot pronounce a product's ingredients and the label sounds more like the supply list for a high school chemistry lab experiment, don't buy the product. A bad grade in chemistry or a burning lab is easier to remedy than your body's ill health.

Orange peel

The food dye citrus red #2, used to dye the skin of oranges, has been shown to cause cancer in animals. This food dye is used to make the greenish appearance of

Florida oranges resemble the deep orange of California oranges. Unless you purchase organically grown oranges, we recommend skipping the orange peel in recipes. In addition, since marmalade contains orange peel, always purchase organic varieties. You may want to preserve the inner portion of the peel. Citrus pulp, the white part of the orange peel, may help prevent breast cancer. A little bit of green does not change the taste of oranges and, in fact, the best oranges the authors have tasted were of the dark green variety in the Caribbean.

Refined sugar

A high intake of rapidly absorbed carbohydrates, also known as a high glycemic load or index, has been associated with the development of cancer of the breast and of the upper digestive tract.

Trans fat

"Trans" fats are produced when liquid oil is converted to a semi-solid state by hydrogenation. The FDA has concluded that trans fat is even more harmful than saturated fat. Beginning in 2006 food labels, under "Nutrition Facts," were required to list the amount of trans fat present in products. The *Institute of Medicine* recommends you consume as little trans fat as possible, with an upper limit of two grams per day. The average adult in the United States now consumes 5.8 grams. Food products that contain trans fat include vegetable shortening, some margarines, and snack foods such as cookies and crackers. Diets high in trans fats are correlated with an increased risk of developing prostate (King, 2005) and breast cancers (Voorrips, 2002). One study revealed that the amount of partially hydrogenated fat in a woman's buttocks predicted her susceptibility to develop breast cancer in the future (Kohlmeier, 1997)! Trans fats also cause coronary artery disease and contribute to obesity.

Pickled foods

Countries in which people consume a lot of salted meat and fish and pickled vegetables, for example Korea and Japan, have high rates of stomach cancer.

SMOKED FOODS

Frequent consumption of smoked food has been associated with cancer of the intestinal tract. Smoked meats contain the carcinogen 3-4 benzopyrene. In addition, polycyclic aromatic hydrocarbons (PAHs), known carcinogens, form on the surface of food during the smoking process. If you have a strong craving for a smoky flavor, try adding a small amount of liquid smoke, available at most grocery stores, to your food: it provides the flavor without the PAHs.

NITRATES/NITRITES

An alarming and well-publicized study done between 1980 and 1987 showed a nine-fold increase in the risk of developing leukemia in children who consumed twelve or more hot dogs per month (Peters, 1994). Another study done in 1993 in Denver reported an increased risk of developing brain tumors in children whose mothers consumed more than one to two hot dogs per week while pregnant, and in children who ate more than one to two hot dogs per week (Sarasua, 1994). Similar findings are noted in more recent studies (Huncharek, 2004). Nitrites are used as preservatives in hot dogs and other meat products, such as prepared lunchmeats and bacon. While nitrites can combine with amines in meat to form carcinogenic compounds, no true cause and effect relationship has been documented. Factors other than nitrites could be responsible for the increased risk, such as the nutrients (for example, those in fruits and vegetables) that are **not** being consumed when hot dogs are a big part of the diet.

We recommend minimizing the intake of nitrites and nitrates until more is known about causality. Nitrite-free hot dogs and lunchmeats are available at health food stores and many regular grocery stores. Do not be alarmed by the color of nitrite-free products, which often appear slightly gray, but rather view the lower aesthetic quality as indicative of a more natural product.

BHT/BHA

BHA (butylated hydroxyanisole), a preservative, is possibly carcinogenic to humans, according to IARC, and has been banned in England, Romania, Sweden, and

Australia. BHT (butylated hydroxytoulene) has been shown to cause cancer in animal studies. BHT and BHA are compounds added to foods to preserve fats and oils. They are found in products such as cereals, baked goods, snack foods, chewing gum, potato chips and other dehydrated potato products, meats, and margarines. Since the purpose of these preservatives is to preserve fats and oils, they are found mostly in foods high in fats and oils, foods whose consumption should be minimized for other reasons as well. Though we recommend avoiding BHT and BHA because of their carcinogenic properties, we note that there is some evidence that BHT slows aging in mice!

Potassium bromate

Potassium bromate is a food additive used to increase the volume of bread. It has been shown to cause cancer and has been banned throughout much of the world. It is still used in the United States but its use is becoming less common in California, where foods containing potassium bromate are now required to have a cancer warning on the label.

Food dyes

Several food dyes have been banned. Several are still being studied. A worthy note is that most foods containing artificial colorings are of low nutritional value and you should minimize eating them regardless of concerns about carcinogenicity.

Practical Points

- ❑ Eat five to nine servings of fruits and vegetables per day.
- ❑ Choose organically grown foods when possible. If cost is an issue, review the list of foods that should be purchased only if they have been grown organically.
- ❑ Avoid fast food and think of alternatives; plan ahead.
- ❑ Clean all produce thoroughly.
- ❑ When grilling, marinate meats first, trim fat, and avoid letting the flames touch the meat.
- ❑ Use a fire chimney instead of lighter fluid.
- ❑ Choose baking, roasting, and boiling over broiling, frying, and grilling.
- ❑ Keep plastic out of the microwave.
- ❑ Toss grains and nuts before they become stale; refrigerate nuts and peanut butter.
- ❑ Do not reuse cooking oil.

Resources and Further Online Information

USDA Agricultural Research Service. National Database for Standard Reference

www.ars.usda.gov/services/docs.htm?docid=9673

This is an excellent reference site providing information about the nutritional as well as vitamin and phytochemical contents of many foods.

Nutrition Data

www.nutritiondata.com

This site is extremely comprehensive, including nutritional facts, with graphics, about almost 10,000 food choices, including detailed information labels from foods available at thirty-five fast food establishments. It also allows you to determine the nutrition content of your own recipes.

The Fast Food Nutrition Fact Explorer

www.fatcalories.com

An easy to navigate site that provides information on the nutritional content of foods available at twelve of the most frequented fast food establishments.

How to Understand and Use the Nutritional Facts Label

www.cfsan.fda.gov/~dms/foodlab.html

The U.S. Food and Drug Administration provides this site about how to understand and use the "nutrition facts" label on foods. The information is presented in a clear and understandable fashion.

Consumer Reports' "When Buying Organic Pays (And Doesn't)"

www.consumerreports.org/cro/food/organic-products-206/when-buying-organic-pays-and-doesnt.htm

This interactive Web site lists foods and cosmetics with recommendations about whether you should purchase organic versions, purchase organic versions only if price is not a concern, or purchase non-organic versions.

"Window to My Environment" on lake fish consumption

www.epa.gov/enviro//wme/

The site "Window to My Environment," provided by the EPA, gives information about fish consumption based on the lake fished. Information is accessed by zip code or city.

FDA data on acrylamide concentration in foods
www.oehha.ca.gov/prop65/acrylamideintakefdaappendix.pdf

This site provides FDA data on acrylamide content in foods.

Mix It Up (MN only)
www.mixitupmeals.com

This company allows you to prepare many meals you can later freeze in their facilities and offers to shop and cut up ingredients prior to your arrival.

Seattle Sutton
www.seattlesutton.com/home.asp

Seattle Sutton offers meals, including food for weight loss plans, which can be delivered to your home or office.

Love and Logic
www.loveandlogic.com/

This site provides information and resources on parenting and teaching responsibility, in an easily adopted, empowering, and humorous fashion, while maintaining the dignity of both parents and children. The authors recommend the books and resources listed on this Web site as staples for any parent.

Whole Foods Market
www.wholefoods.com

The Whole Foods Market Web site provides locations of its nationwide network of retail stores. These stores carry a wide variety of foods that are carefully evaluated, both for nutrition, and for lack of unacceptable food ingredients, taking the guesswork out of the equation as consumers search for healthy food choices. A variety of classes are offered as well, many of which are free to the public, on topics from creating a healthy lunchbox to managing your blood sugar. Health and wellness tips, and many recipes, are also offered.

Fresh and Natural Foods (Minnesota and Wisconsin only)
www.freshandnaturalfoods.com

This Web site provides information on store locations, and also offers classes on various nutrition topics.

The WEDGE Natural Foods Co-op (Minnesota only).
www.wedge.coop/

The Wedge Web site contains interesting information discussing organic farming, and has available a free online newsletter.

Good Earth Natural Foods (California only)
www.goodearthnaturalfoods.net

Good Earth Natural Foods, which carries 100 percent produce that is certified organic, was voted Best Health Food Store for three consecutive years in Marin, Sonoma, and Napa counties. A free online newsletter is available.

Sun Organic Farm
www.sunorganicfarm.com

Sun Organic Farm is an online health food store that offers delivery of organic foods and products to your door. A free organic food catalogue can be obtained by calling them toll free at 1-888-269-9888.

ShopByDiet.com
www.shopbydiet.com

Shopbydiet.com is an online health food store that offers products for those on special diets as well as organic foods. Examples include gluten-free, dairy-free, and low-sodium products.

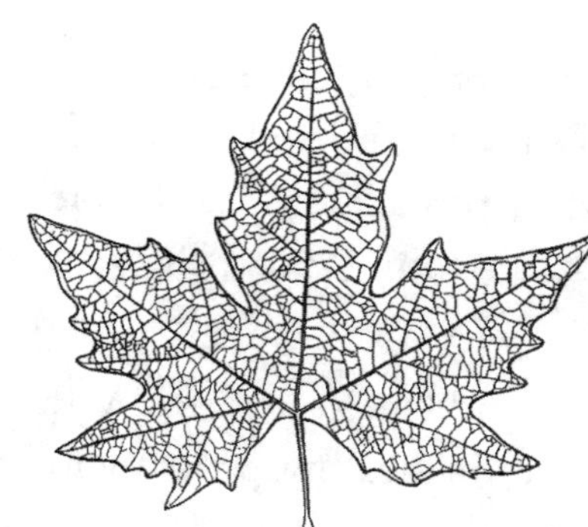

Chapter Nine

Secondary Prevention of Cancer

"A man too busy to take care of his health is like a mechanic too busy to take care of his tools."

—Spanish Proverb

Our emphasis throughout this book has been on the primary prevention of cancer. Despite the vast amount of research, the billions of dollars spent, and the continued development of new technologies and chemotherapy medications, little progress has been made towards decreasing the mortality from cancer. Unless we see unimagined breakthroughs in the near future, and even if we do, primary prevention should remain our first priority.

Secondary prevention is the science of searching for disease in its early stages, when it may be curable. Procedures such as removing precancerous colon polyps and treating abnormal cells on the cervix have been shown to be very beneficial. We believe screening to look for early prostate cancer and breast cancer is important as well, although the impact of this is less clear. There have been some discussions that, through screening, some early cancers are simply picked up at an earlier stage, giving rise to the observed increases in life expectancies. For now, it is important to assume that finding these cancers early does make a difference and to practice the recommended screening guidelines.

In addition to advocating the primary prevention concepts we have discussed at length, we strongly urge our readers to stay up to date on cancer screening and keep a record of tests they have taken. Most people—87 percent in a study published in *JAMA*—believe routine cancer screening is a good idea (Schwarz, 2004). In our clinical practice, we have been surprised at the number of very conscientious people who have neglected their own health maintenance. Most of these people made sure their children were immunized, their cars tuned up, their furnaces inspected, their sprinkler systems blown out, their dogs treated for heartworm, and their smoke detectors working. Make yourself a priority!

Below we list the recommended cancer screening guidelines set forth by the American Cancer Society. These recommendations are for healthy people without symptoms and medical problems or family histories that would indicate cancer risk. Your healthcare provider may recommend additional screening based on concerns he or she may have, given your medical history, family history, and any significant symptoms or findings on exams.

Cancer Screening Guidelines from The American Cancer Society:

The following cancer screening guidelines are recommended for those people at average risk for cancer (unless otherwise specified) and without any specific symptoms.

People who are at increased risk for certain cancers may need to follow a different screening schedule, such as starting at an earlier age or being screened more often. Those with symptoms that could be related to cancer should see their doctor immediately.

Cancer-related checkup

For people having periodic health examinations, a cancer-related checkup should include health counseling and depending on a person's age might include examinations for cancers of the thyroid, oral cavity, skin, lymph nodes, testes, and ovaries as well as for some non-malignant diseases.

The following special tests for certain cancer sites are recommended.

Breast cancer

- Yearly mammograms starting at age 40 and continuing for as long as a woman is in good health.
- Clinical breast exams (CBE) should be part of a periodic health exam, about every three years for women in their 20s and 30s and every year for women 40 and over.
- Women should report any breast change promptly to their healthcare providers. Breast self-exam (BSE) is an option for women starting in their 20s.
- Women at increased risk (e.g., family history, genetic tendency, past breast cancer) should talk with their doctors about the benefits and limitations of starting mammography screening earlier, having additional tests (e.g., breast ultrasound or MRI), or having more frequent exams.

Colon and rectal cancer

Beginning at age 50, both men and women at average risk for developing colorectal cancer should follow one of these five testing schedules:

- yearly fecal occult blood test (FOBT)* or fecal immunochemical test (FIT)
- flexible sigmoidoscopy every 5 years
- yearly FOBT* or FIT plus flexible sigmoidoscopy every 5 years**
- double-contrast barium enema every 5 years
- colonoscopy every 10 years

*For FOBT, the take-home multiple sample method should be used.
**The combination of yearly FOBT or FIT plus flexible sigmoidoscopy every 5 years is preferred over either of these options alone.

All positive tests should be followed up with colonoscopy.

People should begin colorectal cancer screening earlier and/or undergo screening more often if they have any of the following colorectal cancer risk factors:

- a personal history of colorectal cancer or adenomatous polyps
- a strong family history of colorectal cancer or polyps (cancer or polyps in a first-degree relative younger than 60 or in two first-degree relatives of any age). Note: a first degree relative is defined as a parent, sibling, or child.
- a personal history of chronic inflammatory bowel disease
- a family history of a hereditary colorectal cancer syndrome (familial adenomatous polyposis or hereditary non-polyposis colon cancer)

Cervical cancer

The American Cancer Society recommends:

- All women should begin cervical cancer screening about 3 years after they begin having vaginal intercourse, but no later than when they are 21 years old. Screening should be done every year with the regular Pap test or every 2 years using the newer liquid-based Pap test.
- Beginning at age 30, women who have had 3 normal Pap test results in a row may be screened every 2 to 3 years with either the conventional (regular) or liquid-based Pap test. Women who have certain risk factors such as diethylstilbestrol (DES) exposure before birth, HIV infection, or a weakened immune system due to organ transplant, chemotherapy, or chronic steroid use should continue to be screened annually.
- Another reasonable option for women over 30 is to be screened every 3 years (but not more frequently) with either the conventional or liquid-based Pap test, *plus* the HPV DNA test.
- Women 70 years of age or older who have had 3 or more normal Pap tests in a row and no abnormal Pap test results in the last 10 years may choose to stop having cervical cancer screening. Women with a history of cervical cancer, DES exposure before birth, HIV infection or a weakened immune system should continue to have screening as long as they are in good health.

- Women who have had a total hysterectomy (removal of the uterus and cervix) may also choose to stop having cervical cancer screening, unless the surgery was done as a treatment for cervical cancer or pre-cancer. Women who have had a hysterectomy without removal of the cervix should continue to follow the guidelines above.

Endometrial (uterine) cancer

The American Cancer Society recommends that all women should be informed about the risks and symptoms of endometrial cancer, and strongly encouraged to report any unexpected bleeding or spotting to their doctors. For women with or at high risk for hereditary nonpolyposis colon cancer (HNPCC), annual screening should be offered for endometrial cancer with endometrial biopsy beginning at age 35.

Prostate cancer

Both the prostate-specific antigen (PSA) blood test and digital rectal examination (DRE) should be offered annually, beginning at age 50, to men who have at least a 10-year life expectancy. Men at high risk (African-American men and men with a family of one or more first-degree relatives (father, brothers) diagnosed at an early age) should begin testing at age 45. Men at even higher risk, due to multiple first-degree relatives affected at an early age, could begin testing at age 40. Depending on the results of this initial test, no further testing might be needed until age 45.

Information should be provided to all men about what is known and what is uncertain about the benefits and limitations of early detection and treatment of prostate cancer so that they can make an informed decision about testing.

Men who ask their doctor to make the decision on their behalf should be tested. Discouraging testing is not appropriate. Also, not offering testing is not appropriate.

Source: American Cancer Society. American Cancer Society Guidelines for the Early Detection of Cancer. Available at http://www.cancer.org/docroot/PED/content/PED_2_3X_ACS_Cancer_Detection_Guidelines_36.asp.

Resources And further Online Information

National Cancer Institute (NCI) Cancer Screening Overview

www.cancer.gov/cancertopics/screening

The NCI discusses the screening of specific cancer types and provides information for patients and healthcare professionals. The Web site also provides links to sites discussing more specific types of screening, such as that for tumor markers.

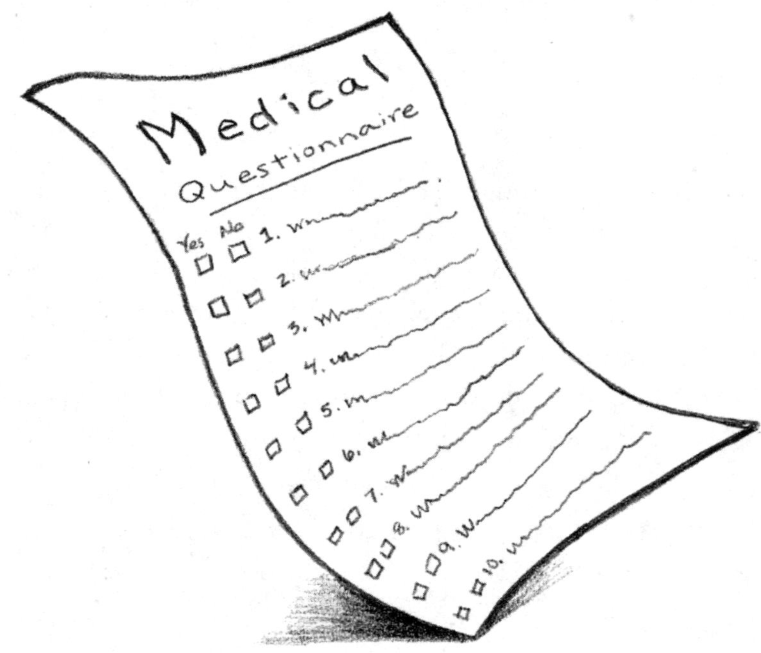

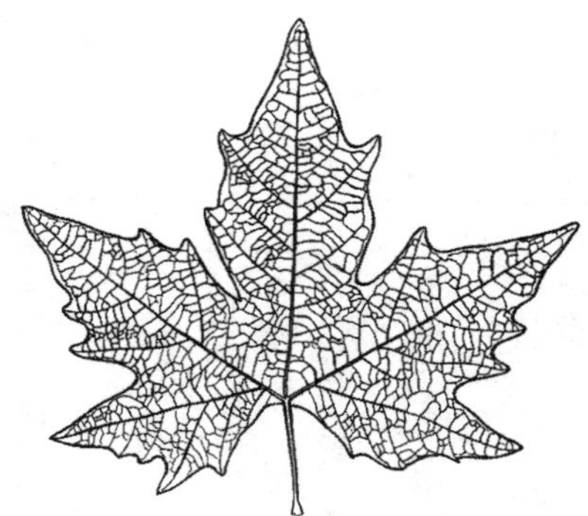

Chapter Ten

Avoiding Cancer Recipe Collection

"Cooking is at once child's play and adult joy. And, cooking done with care is an act of love."

—Craig Clairborne

These recipes are contributed by the authors and our health-conscious friends and family members. We hope that a few of these will please your palate and your lifestyle. Some are contributed by friends with culinary expertise and access to wonderful ingredients, others by those who have limited time and virtually no access to organic ingredients or fresh food. Several are from family and friends who have lost loved ones to cancer, or who have struggled with cancer themselves.

Conversion table for our recipes:
An ounce of prevention is worth a pound of cure.

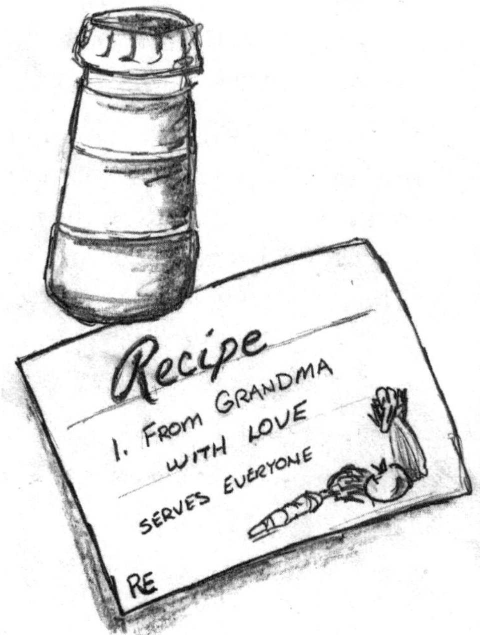

Appetizers and Dips

Crab with Capers

Contributed by Dan Oberdorfer, Minneapolis, Minnesota, good friend of one of the authors

When Dan serves this for company, he prepares the dish up to the addition of the crabmeat and leaves just a little extra liquid. He then reheats the vegetables and adds the crabmeat just before serving.

2 tablespoons olive oil
1 medium onion (chopped)
1 small can Roma tomatoes (chopped to bite-sized pieces)
2 bay leaves
2 heaping teaspoons of sliced, pickled jalapeno slices (or to taste)
2 tablespoons small capers
3 tablespoons large capers
1 pound lump crabmeat
1 small handful Italian parsley leaves (chopped fine)
lime wedges for garnish

In a medium-sized skillet, heat the oil over medium heat. Add the onion and cook until translucent, about 3 minutes. Add the tomatoes and the bay leaves. Cook, stirring occasionally, until the mixture is concentrated, for about 3 or 4 minutes. Add the pickled jalapenos and capers. Cook, stirring occasionally, until most of the liquid has evaporated. Add the crabmeat and cook until heated through, about 2 or 3 minutes. The dish is plenty rich, but you may add a few tablespoons of butter to make it even richer.

Remove the bay leaf and serve with the parsley and lime wedges. This dish makes an excellent appetizer. It may also be used as a filling for tortillas.

This recipe is adapted from *Zarela's Veracruz*, by Zarela Martinez with Anne Mendelson.

HEATHER'S FRESH SALSA

Contributed by Heather Heckman, Hugo, Minnesota, dear friend of one of the authors

Fresh vegetables from the farmer's market make this a summer highlight!

3 to 4 ripe tomatoes, finely chopped
1 green pepper, finely chopped
3 scallions, finely chopped
1 jalapeno pepper, seeded and finely chopped
2 to 3 cloves garlic, pressed
1 teaspoon salt
3 tablespoons lime juice
2 to 3 tablespoons cilantro, chopped

Mix prepared ingredients. Let set for 15 to 20 minutes before serving.

JULIE'S HUMMUS

Contributed by Julie Russell, Shoreview, Minnesota, mother of the authors

This recipe is loaded with "super-foods" for cancer prevention including beans, olive oil, citrus, onion, and Tahini (ground sesame seeds).

1 can (15 ounces) chick peas (garbanzo beans), drained
3 tablespoons onion, finely chopped
1 medium lemon, squeezed, and seeds removed
2 tablespoons olive oil
¼ cup Tahini (ground sesame seeds/sesame paste)
1 clove garlic, pressed (garlic lovers can add another ½ to 1 clove of garlic)
¼ teaspoon sea salt
½ teaspoon ground cumin
freshly ground pepper to taste

Puree above ingredients in a blender or food processor. Serve with sliced cucumbers and slices of whole wheat pita bread.

BREADS/GRAINS

FLAX SEED BREAD (FOR BREAD MACHINES)

The late Helen Russell, grandmother of the authors, developed this recipe. Helen was an RN who worked with Sister Kinney during the polio epidemic, but always had time for her children and grandchildren

Flax is rich in omega-3 fatty acids, which help lower cholesterol. It is also high in lignans, a phytoestrogen that may help prevent breast cancer.

1 ¼ cups water
2 tablespoons honey
2 tablespoons olive oil
1 cup whole wheat bread flour
1 cup unbleached white bread flour
⅓ cup whole flax seed (we prefer the whole flax seed over ground flax for the crunchy flavor)
1 ½ teaspoon salt
2 teaspoons active dry yeast
1 tablespoon poppy seeds
1 tablespoon sesame seeds

Place above ingredients in the order listed in bread maker and bake using the regular cycle. Allow bread to cool before slicing.

BLUEBERRY AND RASPBERRY MUFFINS

Timothy Eldridge, Shoreview, Minnesota, son of one of the authors

When Timmy is not swimming, fishing, riding his bike, or attending his elementary school, he enjoys creating "cancer-prevention" recipes.

1 cup whole wheat flour
½ cup rolled oats
½ cup cornmeal
⅓ cup sugar or honey

1 teaspoon baking powder
1 teaspoon baking soda
¼ teaspoon salt
¼ cup orange juice
2 tablespoons canola oil
½ teaspoon almond extract
1 8-ounce container vanilla yogurt
1 egg
½ cup fresh or frozen organic raspberries
½ cup fresh or frozen organic blueberries

Preheat oven to 400° F. Place paper muffin cups in muffin pan, or spray lightly with olive oil (extra virgin olive oil can be place in a new, prewashed, non-aerosol container for this purpose). In a large bowl, combine dry ingredients. In a second bowl, whisk together orange juice, canola oil, almond extract, yogurt and egg. Combine the wet ingredients with the dry and mix only until moistened. Fold in berries. Divide the batter into muffin cups. Bake until golden brown, about 16 minutes. Remove and let cool before eating. To make these even more appealing to picky eaters, drizzle with a glaze of roughly equal parts powdered sugar and water.

Soups

Grandma Soup

Contributed by Dan Oberdorfer, Minneapolis, Minnesota, friend of one of the authors

Dan would be the envy of any gourmet cook and introduced one of the authors to tasty seaweed. Dan says, "My grandma made this soup, which I think she made up. She added a generous portion of cream and butter, but this is not necessary."

8 large carrots (peeled, trimmed and cut into 4-inch pieces)
3 medium red potatoes (peeled and quartered)
1 parsnip (peeled)
3 celery stalks (cut into 4-inch pieces)
1 medium onion (quartered and skin removed)
2 bay leaves

Place the ingredients in a large pot, and cover with water. Boil until all the vegetables are soft, about 20 minutes. Remove the bay leaves. Celery can be stringy, and may be removed. Puree in a food processor or blender. Add salt and pepper to taste.

Nine Bean Soup

Lynne Eldridge

This recipe includes four beans listed in the USDA list of the top twenty antioxidants. Soaking the beans overnight helps to prevent gas or bloating. This recipe was the authors' grandfather's favorite. At age ninety-one, he would drive over, bringing dinner to me after a long day at work! As our grandparents got older I would bring them dinner, and discovered many healthy recipes that could be prepared ahead of time. This recipe freezes well for easy weekday meals.

⅔ cup dried small red beans
⅔ cup dried red kidney beans
⅓ cup dried pinto beans
⅓ cup dried black beans
⅓ cup dried split peas

⅓ cup lentils
⅓ cup dried garbanzo beans
⅓ cup dried large lima beans
⅓ cup dried black eyed peas
2 cups diced carrots
2 cups diced bokchoy
1 bay leaf
3 cups chopped onions
3 teaspoons sugar
2 teaspoons thyme
5 cloves minced garlic
1 large ham bone
10 teaspoons chicken bouillon granules
5 quarts water
2 teaspoons savory
salt and pepper to taste

Combine beans, peas, and lentils, and rinse thoroughly. Soak in water overnight. Cook ham bone in water in a large Dutch oven 2-3 hours. Let broth cool and skim off all fat. Combine drained beans, peas, and lentils with remaining ingredients, add to broth and simmer 2-3 hours. Remove bay leaf prior to serving.

FARMER'S MARKET SOUP

Lynne Eldridge

This soup makes it easy to add servings of fruits and vegetables to your daily tally, and can serve as a meal or a tasty appetizer. When I prepare this, people usually think from the rich taste that it is loaded with cream and butter.

1 medium onion, chopped
1 clove garlic, minced
¼ cup green pepper, chopped
1 tablespoon butter or olive oil
2 to 3 medium zucchini, sliced (do not peel)
2 apples, peeled and chopped
4 teaspoons chicken base
4 cups water
2 ½ teaspoons curry powder
fresh cilantro, optional

In a large saucepan, sauté onion, garlic, and green pepper in butter or olive oil until tender. Add remaining ingredients except the cilantro and bring to a full boil. Reduce heat and simmer for an additional 20 minutes. Allow soup to cool. In two separate batches, puree soup in blender. Reheat prior to serving and garnish with cilantro.

SALADS

SPINACH-STRAWBERRY SALAD WITH HONEY DRESSING

Contributed by Nancy Johnson, New Brighton, Minnesota. Nancy is the authors' cousin and author of ***Adventure in Dying****, her touching account of her first husband's struggle with cancer. Lin Karo was a healthy pastor only thirty-three years old when he passed away from lymphoma.*

one bag of small organic spinach leaves
Dressing:
½ cup sugar
1 teaspoon dry mustard
1 teaspoon paprika
1 tablespoon lemon juice
1 ½ teaspoons grated onion
1 teaspoon celery salt
⅓ cup honey
5 tablespoons vinegar
1 cup canola oil

Mix dry ingredients. Place in blender. Add honey, vinegar, and lemon juice. Slowly add oil while blending. Top spinach with fresh strawberries and add dressing as desired. Optional: top with hard-boiled eggs or green onions.

Fruit and Herb Salad

Lynne Eldridge and David Borgeson

This recipe is in memory of our father, John Borgeson, who passed away from cancer too young, when he was still able to hike and climb mountains with us.

organic herb greens, or organic baby mixed greens
grapefruit, sectioned
oranges, sectioned
kiwi, peeled and sliced
red grapes, sliced
broccoli sprouts
sunflower seeds
sliced almonds
Dressing:
⅓ cup honey
⅓ cup canola oil
⅓ cup frozen lemonade, from concentrate

Combine honey, oil, and lemonade and blend. Chill for at least 2 hours. Cover individual salad plates with greens. Arrange fruit tastefully over the greens. Top with broccoli sprouts and sprinkle with sesame seeds and sliced almonds. Drizzle with dressing to taste and serve.

Crowd-Pleaser Salad

Contributed by Julie Russell, Shoreview, Minnesota, mother of the authors

This dressing ensures people will have a healthy appetite for leafy greens.

spinach
romaine lettuce
2 large cans mandarin oranges
12 ounces fresh mushrooms, sliced
Dressing:
½ cup sugar

2 tablespoons green onion, chopped
¼ cup white vinegar
¾ cup canola oil
¼ cup extra virgin olive oil
1 teaspoon dried mustard
1 teaspoon salt
1 teaspoon celery seed (important)
2 teaspoons dill weed

Prepare dressing ahead and chill at least 2 hours. Mix equal parts romaine and spinach in a large salad bowl. Toss with mandarin oranges, mushrooms, and dressing to taste just before serving. This dressing stores well and makes a tasty quick meal or snack with an assortment of lettuces.

Rural Fruit Salad

Contributed by Katy Decker, Gwinner, North Dakota, cousin and good friend of the authors

Katy understands that it is still possible to eat healthy despite living in rural Nowhereville, far from any organic or health food stores, or any stores, for that matter!

1 can organic pineapple chunks, drained
2 cans organic tropical fruit salad, drained
Mix, and enjoy.

Nancy's Salad

Contributed by Nancy Johnson, New Brighton, Minnesota, cousin of the authors

romaine lettuce, organic
French dressing:
½ cup sugar
1 ½ teaspoons paprika
1 tablespoon dry mustard
¾ cup canola oil
½ cup vinegar, red wine vinegar, cider vinegar, or balsamic vinegar

Add apple slices or mandarin orange slices. Chicken can also be added.

MAIN DISHES

GRILLED SALMON WITH TERIYAKI SHITAKE

Contributed by Dan Oberdorfer, Minneapolis, Minnesota, good friend of the authors

This recipe combines the cancer- and heart disease-fighting omega-3 fatty acids of salmon, with the powerful antioxidant L-ergothionene found in shiitake mushrooms in a dish that made me want to break the portion law when he prepared it for us!

This recipe is adapted from one of Dr. Andrew Weil's recipes from the February 2006 issue of Food and Wine.

¼ cup sake
2 ½ tablespoons soy sauce
2 ½ teaspoons light brown sugar
2 teaspoons sesame oil
1 tablespoon canola oil
¾ pound shitake mushrooms, stemmed and caps thickly sliced
4 small salmon fillets
1 tablespoon chopped chives or parsley

Pre-heat broiler. Mix the sake, soy sauce, brown sugar and sesame oil in a small bowl. In a large skillet over medium heat, heat half of the canola oil and add the mushrooms over medium heat, stirring occasionally until lightly browned and tender, about 8 minutes. Over high heat, add the sake mixture and cook until the mixture is reduced by half (when serving for company, this dish can be prepared ahead until this point). Remove the mushrooms from the pan, and add the rest of the canola oil. Heat, and then add the salmon filets. Cook over high heat, turning once, until lightly browned, for about 4 minutes.

Place salmon in a heat-proof pan and broil the salmon until golden brown. Return the salmon to the stovetop, return the mushrooms to the pan and cook over high heat until the liquid is evaporated and the salmon and mushrooms have begun to caramelize.

Garnish with chives or parsley and serve.

Baked Tilapia

Contributed by Sharon Alberg, Deephaven, Minnesota, friend of the authors

3 tilapia filets
parsley (1 teaspoon dried or 2 tablespoons chopped)
1 egg
¼ cup grated parmesan cheese
¼ cup whole wheat cracker crumbs (such as My Family Farm® whole wheat baked crackers—animal crackers)
⅓ cup shredded parmesan cheese

Preheat oven to 400° F. Mix together cracker crumbs, grated parmesan cheese, and parsley in a small, rectangular dish. In another small dish, whisk the egg. Spray a cookie sheet or pizza pan with olive oil. Dip each piece of fish into the egg and then the crumb mixture. Place on cookie sheet. Sprinkle fish with shredded parmesan cheese. Bake for 20 minutes. Serve with lemon and/or melted butter.

Serve with brown rice, baked potato, or roasted potato with broccoli

Spaghetti with Meatballs

Contributed by Julie Russell, Shoreview, Minnesota, mother of the author,

This recipe easily disguises a whole head of cauliflower amidst ingredients children will usually eat. Thanks, Mom!

Sauce:

3 8-ounce cans organic tomato sauce
1 12-ounce can organic tomato paste
1 28-ounce can organic whole tomatoes
1 large onion (chopped finely)
1 head of cauliflower (very finely chopped)
2 cloves garlic
1 ½ teaspoons salt
¼ teaspoon nutmeg
1 ½ tablespoons oregano

1 teaspoon thyme
1 tablespoon sugar
3 tablespoons olive oil
Combine ingredients and simmer for 3 hours.

Meatballs:

1 pound ground buffalo (may substitute organic, hormone-free beef or ground turkey)
¼ cup bread crumbs
1 beaten egg
1 clove garlic
¼ cup organic parmesan cheese
1 tsp salt

After simmering sauce for 3 hours, add meatballs and simmer at least 30 minutes, until meat is thoroughly cooked. Serve garnished with mushrooms, parsley, and parmesan cheese, as desired. Do not let children know there is cauliflower in this recipe unless they are fond of vegetables!

Special Chicken with Rice

Contributed by Nancy Johnson, New Brighton, Minnesota, cousin of the authors

1 whole free-range chicken
1 ½ cups brown rice
¼ cup cornstarch
1 ½ cups green pepper, coarsely chopped
3 tablespoons lite soy sauce
¾ cup onions, thinly sliced
2 cups chicken pieces, reserved from chicken
3 tablespoons canola oil
3 ripe tomatoes, cut into thin wedges

Boil chicken and reserve stock. Cut chicken into bite-sized pieces to make 2 cups and set aside. Prepare rice according to package directions. Keep warm. Meanwhile, cook green pepper and onions in heated oil in covered skillet over low heat until tender but not browned. Blend cornstarch with a small amount of chicken stock, add remaining stock and soy sauce. Gently stir chicken and stock into vegetables. Cook and stir until sauce is clear and thickened. Add tomatoes and cook just until heated. Serve over warm rice.

Almond Stir-Fry

Contributed by Katy Decker, Gwinner, North Dakota, cousin and friend of the authors

1 tablespoon canola oil
1 cup cauliflower or broccoli
½ pound carrots
½ pound fresh green beans
4 green onions
1 sweet red pepper
1 cup hot water
1 chicken bouillon cube or 1 teaspoon bouillon granules
2 teaspoons cornstarch
1 2 ¼-ounce package of sliced almonds

Slice carrots into thin strips; trim green beans into 1-inch pieces; slice green onions; and cut red pepper into thin strips for cooking. Heat oil in wok or skillet over medium heat for 1 minute. Add carrot slices and beans and cook for 5 minutes. Add cauliflower, green onions, and red pepper and stir-fry for 4 more minutes. Combine water, cornstarch, and bouillon, stirring until smooth. Add combination to stir-fry, stirring constantly for about 3 minutes or until thickened. Add almonds and stir-fry for approximately an additional minute. Serves 4.

For variety, chicken can be added to this recipe.

Venison Pepper Steak

Contributed by Karen Klefsas, Blaine, Minnesota, dear friend of one of the authors

Karen shares this recipe in loving memory of her husband, Thomas Klefsas, who passed away with pancreatic cancer in April of 2005. This was one of his favorite recipes.

Karen, it was just yesterday we went through pregnancies together. In honor of Pam and Amy I promise we will continue in our search for what causes cancer and how we can prevent it.

1 ½ pounds venison or hormone-free round steak
1 green pepper
1 onion
2 teaspoons beef bouillon
2 tablespoons cornstarch

Cut up venison into bite-sized pieces and place in a pan. Dice up green pepper and onion and add to the pan. Cover with water and add bouillon. Simmer 1 ½ hours until tender. Dissolve cornstarch in ¼ cup water, place in pan, and stir until thickened.

Supersize Turkey Spinach Meatballs

Contributed by Heather Heckman, Hugo, Minnesota, friend of one of the authors

Heather and Lynne share a passion to fill their children with healthy vegetables, sometimes by creatively disguising them. Heather's kids love this recipe!

1 10-ounce package frozen chopped spinach
2 ½ pounds ground turkey
½ medium onion, chopped
3 garlic cloves, pressed
1 large egg
¼ cup milk
¾ cup bread crumbs (dried whole wheat bread)
½ cup freshly grated parmesan cheese
kosher salt and freshly ground pepper to taste

Preheat oven to 400° F. Cook and dry spinach. Place ground turkey in a large bowl and make a large well in the middle. Add remainder of ingredients to the well, and mix until combined. Form mixture into 12 large balls and arrange on a baking sheet. Drizzle with extra virgin olive oil. Roast for 25 minutes until cooked through and warm.

Serve over spinach egg noodles with green salad.

Salmon-Stuffed Tomatoes

Contributed by Julie Russell, Shoreview, Minnesota, mother of the authors

Salad:

1 ½ cups wild rice, cooked and chilled
1 15-ounce can salmon, drained and flaked
½ cup carrots, shredded
½ cup green onions, sliced
½ cup cucumbers, seeded and chopped

Dressing:

½ cup sour cream (may substitute ½ cup plain yogurt)
4 teaspoons juice
2 tablespoons fresh dill, chopped (may substitute 2 teaspoons dried dill weed)
¼ teaspoon salt
4 large tomatoes

Combine salad ingredients in a large bowl and toss gently. In a small bowl, combine dressing ingredients and mix well with a wire whisk. Core tomatoes and slice into sixths, maintaining the bottom to create a bowl. Fill tomatoes with salad and dressing mixture and serve.

PITA BREAD SANDWICHES

Lynne Eldridge

This is Jessica's favorite; children tend to eat more vegetables when they are "hidden" in a pocket.

whole wheat organic pita bread
plain yogurt
turkey slices, nitrate-free
cucumber slices
apple slices
broccoli sprouts
romaine lettuce
tomato slices

Lightly toast pita bread. Spread inside of pocket with yogurt. Fill pocket with an assortment of the above ingredients, or add your own ideas and seasonal vegetables. Drizzle with olive oil and serve.

VEGETABLE SIDE DISHES

PLANKED MEDITERRANEAN VEGETABLES

Contributed by Christine Altenhoffen, Shoreview, Minnesota, dear friend of one of the authors

This recipe is dedicated in memory of Christine's late husband Michael Altenhoffen. Michael was a marathoner and his healthy habits showed in his vibrant smile. He passed away from lymphoma at the young age of 37, leaving behind an adoring wife and three beautiful children.

¼ cup olive oil
3 tablespoons balsamic vinegar
1 tablespoon Dijon mustard

1 tablespoon honey
2 zucchini, cut into 1-inch cubes
2 yellow squash, cut into 1-inch cubes
1 red onion, cut into 1-inch pieces
1 cup baby carrots
8-ounces button mushrooms, halved
5 cloves garlic, coarsely chopped
10 cherry tomatoes
¼ cup fresh mixed herbs, chopped (basil, rosemary, and chives)
salt and pepper
½ cup feta cheese, crumbled
2 15-inch soaked cedar, maple, or alder grilling planks

Preheat grill to 350° F. Combine oil, balsamic vinegar, mustard, and honey in a small bowl; pour over vegetables (zucchini through garlic) and toss gently. Sprinkle with salt and pepper. Place two soaked planks on hot grill and close lid. Heat planks for 5 minutes or until light smoke develops. Spread vegetables on hot planks and grill over indirect heat for approximately 20 minutes, until vegetables are almost done. Add cherry tomatoes to vegetables and grill 2-3 minutes until vegetables are tender. Remove vegetables from grill and place in large bowl. Gently toss with fresh herbs, salt and pepper, and feta cheese.

—Serves 6-8

Cedar planks can be purchased at discount stores such as Target or gourmet specialty shops. Christine makes this recipe more budget-friendly by preparing her own cedar planks. At Home Depot she purchases cedar fence planks—untreated of course. A single piece of cedar cut at fifteen-inch intervals provides five planks. She then sands these down slightly. She cautions that these require more time to soak and can burn a little on the bottom. Keep a spray bottle handy to put out any fires.

Sesame Kale

Lynne Eldridge

Kale is high in lutein, which is becoming recognized for its role in preventing the development of cancer and the clearance of cancer-causing viruses. It also has a role in delaying the development of cataracts and macular degeneration. This recipe also includes garlic, seaweed, and sesame oil for their anticancer properties. Use organic sesame seeds to minimize pesticide residue.

1 pound kale (or 1 bunch)
2 cloves garlic (minced)
2 teaspoons sesame seed oil
2 tablespoons water
1 teaspoon lite soy sauce
2 teaspoons toasted organic sesame seeds
⅛ cup dried seaweed (optional)

Prepare seaweed per package directions. Mince garlic cloves. Wash kale and tear into bite size pieces keeping it somewhat wet. Heat sesame oil over medium temperature. Add garlic and sauté until lightly browned. Add kale, seaweed, water and soy sauce and cook until kale is wilted, approximately 2 minutes. Add sesame seeds and serve. This recipe is excellent served chilled as well.

Broccoli and Sesame Seeds

Contributed by Kathleen Freeman, Vadnais Heights, Minnesota, good friend of one of the authors

Kathleen contributed this recipe in memory of her late husband, Bruce Miller, who left this world and their young son far too early with ampullary cancer. Katherine showed us her great inner strength and dedication as she cared for Bruce, and through witnessing her caring ways, Bruce's life has touched many.

1 pound broccoli
2 tablespoons sesame seeds
2 tablespoons slivered almonds
1 tablespoon sesame oil

1 tablespoon flax oil (1 tablespoon sesame oil or olive oil may be substituted)
kosher salt

Clean broccoli and cut into florets. Cut off the bottom inch of stems, peel stems, and cut into thin pieces. Add sesame oil and flax oil to a medium sized-skillet. Over medium-high heat sauté sesame seeds and almond slices until light golden brown, around 2-3 minutes. Steam broccoli until tender, for about 7 minutes. Transfer to a large bowl and toss with sesame almond mixture. Season to taste with kosher salt and serve warm; or prepare ahead and serve chilled for a refreshing side dish.

Roasted Parsnips

Contributed by Dan Oberdorfer, Minneapolis, Minnesota, good friend of one of the authors

2 pounds parsnips (peeled and sliced into 4-inch pieces)
2 tablespoons olive oil
salt to taste

Preheat oven to 500° F.

Coat the parsnips with the olive oil and salt. If you like, you may add fresh herbs such as rosemary, thyme, or parsley. Mix together, then roast the parsnips in the oven for about 30 minutes, turning once, until golden brown. To enhance caramelization, add a little brown sugar to the parsnips.

You may use the same recipe with most vegetables, including potatoes, fennel, leaks, beets, or carrots. Cooking times vary.

Roasted Onion Potatoes

Contributed by Sharon Alberg, Deephaven, Minnesota, good friend of the authors

4 medium-sized red or Yukon gold potatoes
½ package organic onion soup mix
¼ cup olive oil

Cut potatoes into 8 pieces (about ¾ inch). Place olive oil and soup mix in a zip-lock bag. Add potatoes and shake well. Remove potatoes and place on cookie sheet. Bake for 40 minutes at 400° F.

Beverages

Triple-Berry Smoothie

Lynne Eldridge

The children's favorite and simple enough that we make it often.

3 cups organic frozen berries (blueberries, strawberries, raspberries, marionberries)
8 large ice cubes
1 cup skim milk (from cows not treated with BST)
¼ cup sugar

Mix above ingredients and blend until the desired consistency.

FRUIT SMOOTHIE

Contributed by Sharon Alberg, Deephaven, Minnesota, good friend of the authors

Sharon has been a good friend to both authors for many years and was designing cancer-prevention recipes using organic ingredients long before "organic" became a popular catch-word.

5 ounces frozen fruit
1 frozen banana
2 oranges (sections or slice into quarters and remove orange with grapefruit knife)
1 cup fruit juice
4-8 ounces soy or dairy yogurt (plain or fruit-flavored)
2 scoops (6 tablespoons) protein power (whey or soy protein with Spirulina)
2 tablespoons lecithin Granules (NOW® brand)
2 tablespoons flax oil with lignan
½ to 2 tablespoons brewer's yeast

Place all ingredients in a blender: alternate blending on the highest speed for 30 seconds and pulsating using the ice crush option until smooth. Makes 2 servings (about 12 oz each).

Combinations that work well are:

Frozen mango with orange juice
Frozen peach with orange juice
Frozen mixed berry (strawberry, blueberry, ras pberry) with red raspberry or apple juice
Frozen strawberry with orange or apple juice

Organic ingredients are recommended.

DESSERT

RHUBARB-HICKORY NUT BREAD

Contributed by Lynette Schultz, Webster, Wisconsin, friend of the authors

Lynette dedicates this recipe to her friend and cancer survivor Judy Gietzel-Schnacky, and also to her friend Thelma Ess, who lost her fight with cancer and left us much too soon.

1 cup rhubarb, coarsely chopped
1 cup sugar
1 ½ cup flour
1 ½ teaspoons baking powder
½ teaspoon baking soda
½ teaspoon salt
1 egg
2 tablespoons milk (from cows not treated with BST)
4 tablespoons butter, melted
½ cup hickory nuts, coarsely chopped

Let the rhubarb steep in ½ cup of the sugar for 1 hour or more (even overnight), stirring once or twice. Toss the remaining sugar and all of the dry ingredients together to mix thoroughly. Beat the egg lightly and stir into it ¼ cup of the juice that the rhubarb will have exuded after steeping, as well as the milk and melted butter. Mix the dry indredients into the wet, stirring just enough to mix. Fold in the rhubarb (if there is still more juice, drain it off) and the nuts. Scrape the batter into a buttered 8-inch loaf pan and bake in a preheated 350° F oven for 1 hour. Let the loaf rest in the pan 10 minutes before unmolding, then cool it on a rack.

Simple Sorbet

Contributed by Timothy Eldridge, Shoreview, Minnesota, son of one of the authors

Dessert can be tasty, while still adding to the 5 to 9 list.

2 cups fresh or canned pineapple chunks, frozen
⅓ cup organic raspberries, frozen
⅓ cup organic blueberries, frozen
⅓ cup organic strawberries, sliced and frozen
1 banana, sliced and frozen
1 cup pineapple juice
2 tablespoons pistachios, chopped

Allow frozen fruit to thaw for 10 to 15 minutes. Place all ingredients in blender and blend until smooth. Place mixture in individual cups and sprinkle with pistachios. Serve immediately.

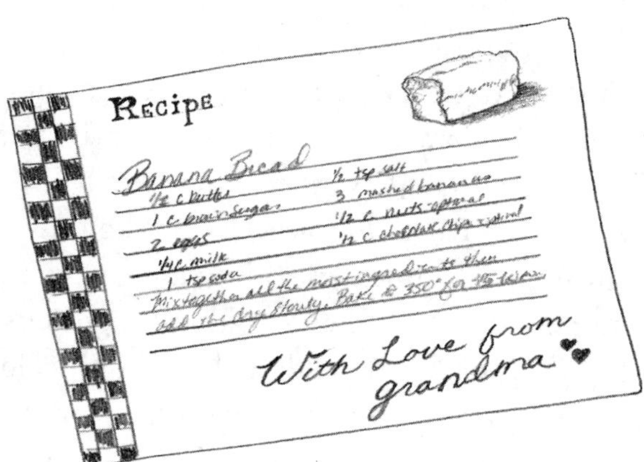

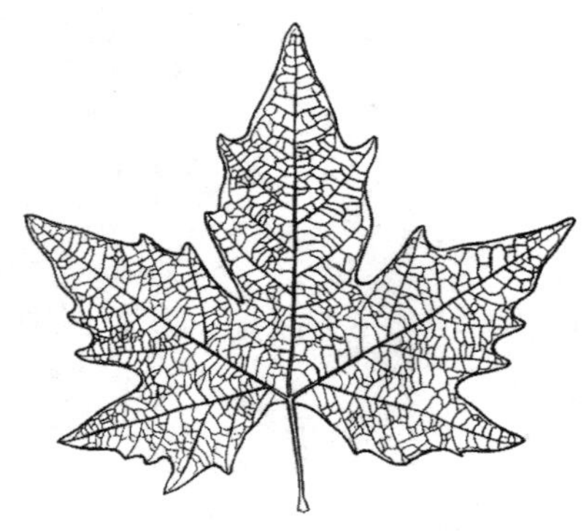

Chapter Eleven

Concluding Remarks

"Take this at least, this last advice, my son:
Keep a stiff rein, and move but gently on:
The coursers of themselves will run too fast,
Your art must be to moderate their haste."

—Ovid (Publicus Ovidus Naso)

Much of what we need to do to prevent cancer comes down to common sense, something that is often overlooked in our rapidly paced, high-tech society. The authors' grandparents, who lived healthy, active lives well into their nineties, practiced many of the principles we seem to have forgotten today. They opened windows to air out their home even in the dead of Minnesota winters. They ate fruits and vegetables religiously at each meal. They purchased produce in-season. Dinners including meat were reserved for Sundays. They encouraged their children and grandchildren to go outside for exercise and sunlight (vitamin D), even on those coldest days. High-calorie foods and soda were special treats. Abstinence before marriage was condoned rather than ridiculed. They carefully turned off lights at night. They respected the sun and limited their time outside during midday, using protective clothing and shelter rather than using chemicals to coat their bodies and erase all cause for concern. Drycleaners were used for wedding dresses and other items, where the expense justified the cost. Everything they ate or wore was prewashed, in case they contained germs or chemicals. They came inside at dusk rather than lathered themselves profusely with bug spray. They did not have the "privilege" of non-stick cookware or access to anything they could want packaged for instant microwave heating. They were suspicious of new medications, products, and fast food. They did not do things to excess, as we are so prone to do now, and they practiced moderation. They seemed to know intuitively when to keep a stiff reign and exhibit caution, and never had a chance to read our book!

There were things they did not understand. They did not have their home checked for radon. They ate out in restaurants filled with secondhand smoke. They stayed warm with the help of asbestos insulation. They painted their home and furniture with lead-based paint. They loved the taste of their well water and never had it tested. Nevertheless, when information about risk became available, they listened.

Some people seem to "get away with" eating too much, smoking and drinking too much, and exposing themselves to carcinogens. Others do not. Our grandparents did not "gamble" with their lives. Through their actions they also demonstrated that life is more than preventing cancer, and we cherish the memories we have of their playfulness, love, and smiles. We have witnessed those who have succumbed to cancer at young ages but who lived life passionately and fully. We have also seen those that lived to ninety without cancer, but who lacked a passion and love of life. This book was designed for those who have that zest of our ancestors, and who hope for a long, full, cancer-free life.

Resources for Further Information on Cancer Prevention

American Cancer Society

www.cancer.org/

The American Cancer Society has a twenty-four hour number and they address nearly any cancer-related topic at 1-800-ACS-2345.

The National Cancer Institute

www.cancer.gov/

The National Cancer Institute provides extensive information based on cancer types, as well as cancer topics and information on clinical trials.

CDC Cancer Prevention and Control

www.cdc.gov/CANCER/

This CDC Web site includes a resource library for cancer, as well as links discussing several cancer topics.

Pubmed

www.ncbi.nlm.nih.gov/entrez/query.fcgi?DB=pubmed.

Pubmed offers links to a multitude of medical journals, many of which provide free abstracts.

Oncolink

www.oncolink.upenn.edu

An excellent Web site provided by the Abramson Cancer Center at the University of Pennsylvania. This site, in addition to providing information on cancer types and treatment, provides the latest news on cancer treatment and prevention. It also provides information on coping for those who have been diagnosed with cancer, including a unique poem-writing feature for cancer patients and their caregivers.

APPENDICES

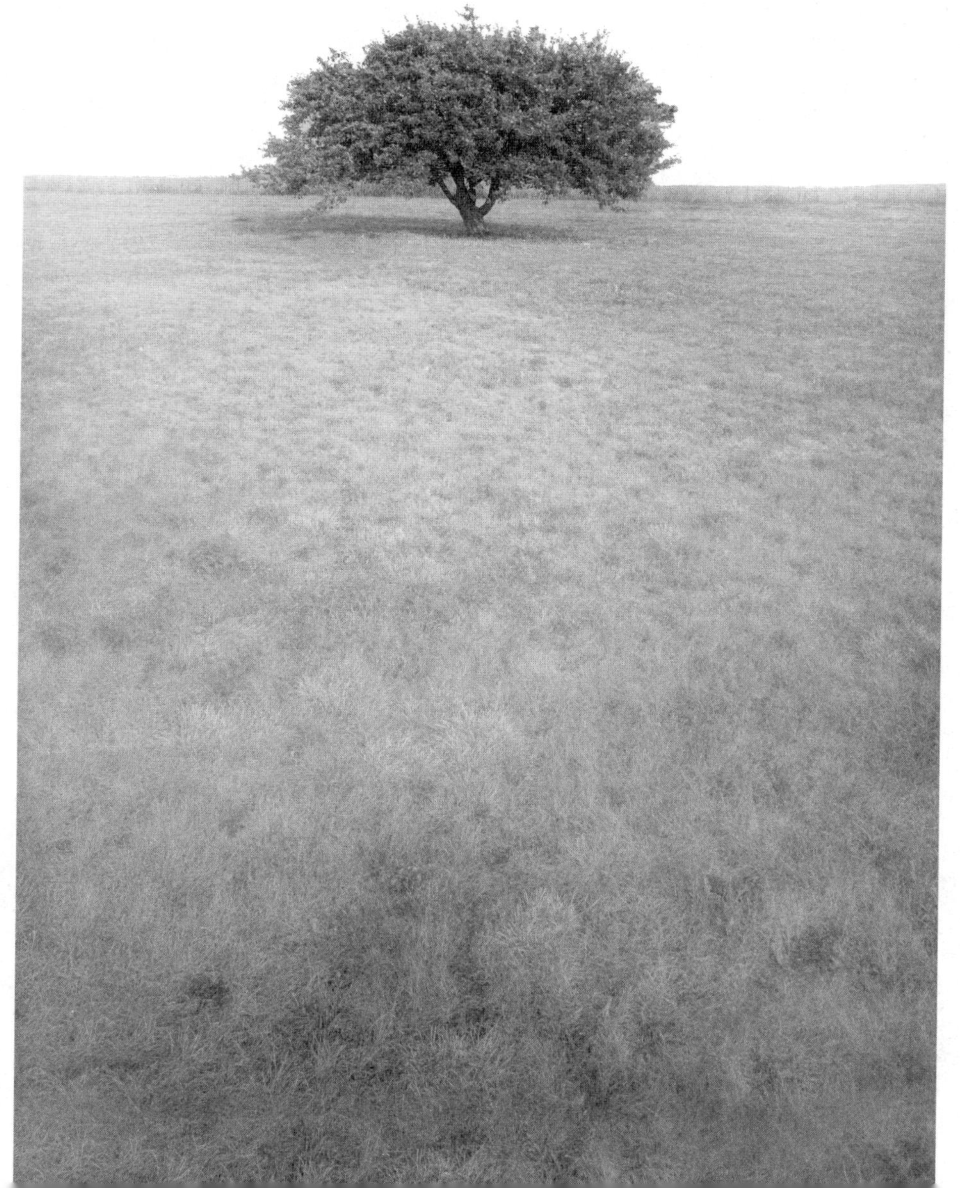

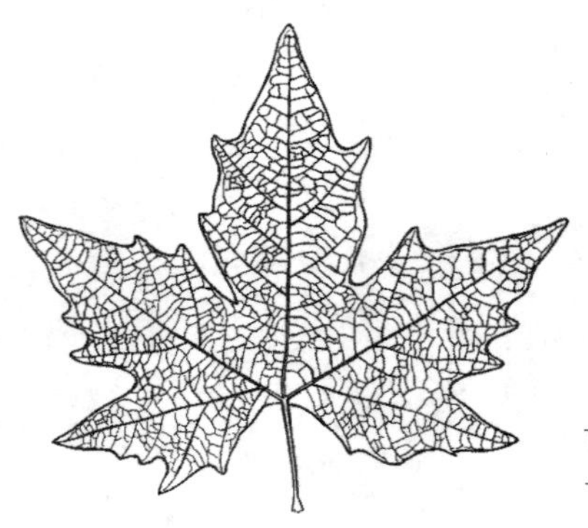

Appendix A

Worksheets For Applying Cancer-Prevention Principles

Radon detection

Kits are available at hardware stores, or through the National Radon Helpline at 1-800-557-2366.

Date tested for radon level in your home: ____________________

Result: ____

____

____

Upper limit of normal: 4pCi/L; average level in U.S. homes: 1.3 pCi/L

For smokers:

Date set for quitting smoking: ____________________________

Assistance available at: www.cancer.org or www.cdc.gov/tobacco/ho22quit.htm.

Family history worksheet:

Family History Cancer Chart

Cancer Type	Age of Onset	Parents	Siblings	Grandparents	Children	Extended Family
Breast						
Colon						
Ovarian						
Lung						
Melanoma						
Other						

Checking your home for carcinogens worksheet:

Cleaning out closets/reading labels with assistance of the carcinogen lists in Appendices B and C

Specific products without ingredients listed can be checked out at http://householdproducts.nlm.nih.gov/products.htm

Date products in your closets and cupboards were evaluated: ________________

Removal of any damaged non-stick pans (check when done): ________________

Shopping list for a safe home

Impermeable gloves (date purchased): ________________

Alternative cleaners such as baking soda, lemon juice, borax, vinegar, cream of tartar, mineral oil, natural soap flakes, steel wool (dates purchased): ______________

Foods to buy only if they are grown or contain ingredients grown organically. Check off when you have switched to these:

Fruits

- ❑ Apples
- ❑ Grapes
- ❑ Peaches
- ❑ Raspberries
- ❑ Cherries
- ❑ Nectarines
- ❑ Pears
- ❑ Strawberries

Vegetables

- ❑ Bell peppers
- ❑ Potatoes
- ❑ Celery
- ❑ Spinach

- ❑ **Beef** (all)
- ❑ **Chicken** (all)

Dairy

- ❑ Milk
- ❑ Baby food (all)
- ❑ Eggs

For those with well water:

Date water was tested: ________________

Results: ____

____

Date filter purchased and type: ____

Maintenance requirements: ____

____

For those exposed to chemicals at work:

Date Material Data Safety Sheets reviewed:________________

List any chemicals or concerns or changes to be made: _______________________

____

If you have an outddor wooden play set constructed prior to 2003:

Date sealed*: ________________

Date soil beneath play set tested, if desired: ________________

*(recommended ideally every six months, but at least annually)

Vaccination history:

Hepatitis B: ________________ ________________ ________________

Recommended for all children, adolescents, and high-risk adults. Ideally received by everyone.

HPV: ________________ ________________ ________________

The HPV vaccine was approved in June 2006 but may not be widely available at the time of printing. It is recommended for girls and women age nine to twenty-six. Women older than twenty-six who are not in monogamous relationships can discuss this with their health-care provider.

Travel diary for infectious agents:

Region to be traveled to: ____

CDC recommendations regarding liver flukes, shistosomiasis, other:

____

____

EXERCISE DIARY

(It takes twenty-one days to establish a habit.)

Day	Exercise Type	Minutes Exercised
1		
2		
3		
4		
5		
6		
7		
8		
9		
10		
11		
12		
13		
14		
15		
16		
17		
18		
19		
20		
21		

Congratulations!

Food diary

List for nine fruits and veggies per day for twenty-one days.

Day	Food Eaten	# Fruits	# Vegetables	TOTAL
1				
2				
3				
4				
5				
6				
7				
8				
9				
10				
11				
12				
13				
14				
15				
16				
17				
18				
19				
20				
21				

If you have gastritis or ulcers:

Date of test for *H. pylori:* ________________ Results: ________________________

Recommendations from your healthcare provider: ____________________________

____

If you have gastroesophageal reflux:

Date of diagnosis: ______________

Date of endoscopy if symptoms have been present for more than five years: ______________

Stress reduction:

Date of discussion with a friend (see page 108): ______________

Changes you will attempt to make in your life (list at least five):

____

____

____

____

____

Resources for management (e.g., yoga, prayer, meditation, exercise): __________

____

Review of sleep patterns and habits:

Dates reviewed: ______________

Average sleep per night: ______________

Changes you may want to consider: ______________

Do you sleep in total darkness?: ______________

Review of body mass index (see Table 6-3):

Result: ______________ Goal: ______________

Changes to reach goal: ______________________________

____

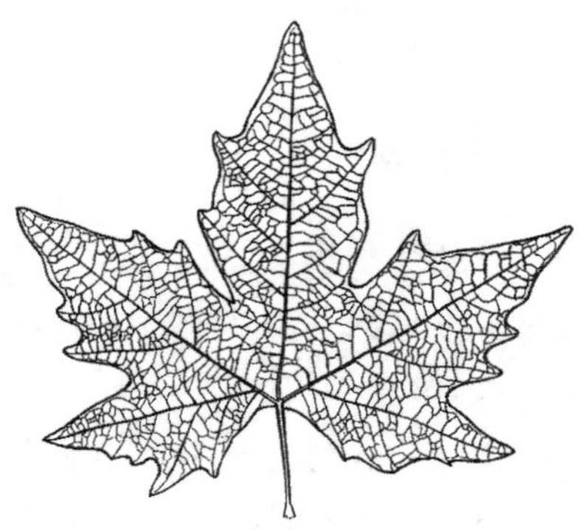

Appendix B

Carcinogen List

Three major lists of carcinogens have been published that classify substances in regard to their ability to cause cancer. If a substance appears on one list but not another, it does not imply a discrepancy in thoughts of carcinogenicity. Different substances have been evaluated by these agencies, and therefore, the list that follows is a compilation of their findings. These include:

The International Agency for Research on Cancer (IARC)

The IARC is part of the World Health Organization, and has classified approximately 900 substances into one of five categories.

- Class 1—Known human carcinogens
- Class 2A—Probable human carcinogens
- Class 2B—Possible human carcinogens
- Class 3—Not classifiable for human carcinogenicity
- Class 4—Probably not carcinogenic to humans

The National Toxicology Program (NTP)

The National Toxicology Program is part of the U.S. Department of Health and Human Services. The NTP provides a report on carcinogens that is updated every two years and classifies substances in two categories.

- NTP-1—Known human carcinogen
- NTP—Reasonably anticipated to be human carcinogen

The Occupational Safety and Health Administration (OSHA)

The Occupational Safety and Health Administration is part of the U.S. Department of Labor. OSHA provides information on carcinogens in the workplace.

The following list is a compilation of carcinogen lists put forth by IARC, NTP, and OSHA that meet the OSHA definition of "Select Carcinogens." This list is adapted from one prepared by the University of Maryland as part of their "Chemical Hygiene Plan."

A-alpha-C(2-amino-9H-pyrido[2,3-beta]indole)
IARC 2B

Acetaldehyde (75-07-0)
IARC 2B, NTP

Acetamide
IARC 2B

2-Acetylaminofluorene
OSHA, NTP

Acrylamide
IARC 2A, NTP

Acrylonitrile
OSHA*, IARC 2B, NTP

Actinomycin D
IARC 2B

Adriamycin
IARC 2A, NTP

AF-2[2-(2-Furyl)-3-(5-nitro-2-furyl)acrylamide]
IARC 2B

Aflatoxins
IARC 1, NTP-1

Aflatoxin M1
IARC 2B

Alcoholic beverages
IARC 1

2-Aminoanthraquinone
NTP

para-Aminoazobenzene
IARC 2B

ortho-Aminoazotoluene
IARC 2B, NTP

4-Aminobiphenyl (4-Aminodiphenyl)
OSHA, IARC 1, NTP-1

1-Amino-2-methylanthraquinone
NTP

2-Amino-1-methyl-6-phenylimidazo-[4,5-b]pyridine (PhIP)
IARC 2B

2-Aminonaphthalene
IARC 1, NTP-1

2-Amino-5-(5-nitro-2-furyl)-1,3,4-thiadiazole
IARC 2B

Amitrole
IARC 2B, NTP

Analgesic mixtures containing phenacetin
IARC 1, NTP-1

Androgenic (Anabolic) steroids
IARC 2A

ortho-Anisidine
IARC 2B

ortho-Anisidine hydrochloride
NTP

Antimony trioxide
IARC 2B

Aramite
IARC 2B

Aroclor (as polychlorinated biphenyls)
NTP

Arsenic and arsenic compounds
OSHA*, IARC 1, NTP-1

Asbestos
OSHA*, IARC 1, NTP-1

Auramine (Technical Grade)
IARC 2B

Azacitidine
IARC 2A, NTP

Azaserine
IARC 2B

Azathioprine
IARC 1, NTP-1

Aziridine
IARC 2B

Benz[a]anthracene
IARC 2A, NTP

Benzene
OSHA*, IARC 1, NTP-1

Benzidine
OSHA, IARC 1, NTP-1

Benzidine-based dyes
IARC 2A, NTP

Benzo[b] fluoranthene
IARC 2B, NTP

Benzo[j] fluoranthene
IARC 2B, NTP

Benzo[k] fluoranthene
IARC 2B, NTP

Benzofuran
IARC 2B

Benzo[a] pyrene
IARC 2A, NTP

Benzotrichloride
NTP

Benzyl violet 4B
IARC 2B

Beryllium & beryllium compounds
IARC 1, NTP

Betel quid with tobacco
IARC 1

N,N-Bis(2-chloroethyl)-2-naphthylamine (Chlornaphazine)
IARC 1

Bischloroethyl nitrosourea (BCNU)
IARC 2A, NTP

Bis(chloromethyl) ether
NTP-1

Bis(chloromethyl) ether and chloromethyl methyl ether (Technical Grade)
OSAH, IARC 1

Bituments, extracts of steam-refined and air-refined
IARC 2B

Bleomycins
IARC 2B

Bracken fern
IARC 2B

Bromodichloromethane
IARC 2B, NTP

Busulfan (1,4-Butanediol Dimethylsulfonate; Myleran)
IARC 1, NTP-1

1,3-Butadiene
IARC 2A, NTP

1,4-butanediol dimethanesulfonate (Busulphan; Myleran)
IARC 1, NTP-1

Butylated hydroxyanisole (BHA)
IARC 2B, NTP

beta-Butyrolactone
IARC 2B

Cadmium and cadmium compounds
OSHA*, IARC 1, NTP

Caffeic acid
IARC 2B

Captafol
IARC 2A

Carbon-black
IARC 2B

Carbon Tetrachloride
IARC 2B, NTP

Carrageenan
IARC 2A

Catechol
IARC 2B

Ceramic fibers (respirable size)
IARC 2B, NTP

Chlorambucil
IARC 1, NTP-1

Chloramphenicol
IARC 2A

Chlordane
IARC 2B

Chlordecone (Kepone)
IARC 2B

Chlorendic acid
IARC 2B, NTP

Chlorinated paraffins (average carbon chain length C12 and average 60% chlorination)
IARC 2B, NTP

alpha-Chlorinated toluenes (combined exposures to benzal chloride, benzotrichloride, benzyl chloride, benzoyl chloride)
IARC 2A

para-Chloroaniline
IARC 2B

1-(2-Chloroethyl)-3-cyclohexyl-1-nitrosourea (CCNU)
IARC 2A, NTP

1-(2-Chloroethyl)-3-(4-methylcyclohexyl)-1-nitrosourea (Methyl-CCNU; Semustine)
IARC 1, NTP-1

Chloroform
IARC 2B, NTP

Chloromethyl methyl ether
NTP-1

1-Chloro-2-methylpropene
IARC 2B

3-Chloro-2-methylpropene
NTP

Chlorophenoxy herbicides
IARC 2B

4-Chloro-ortho-phenylenediamine
IARC 2B, NTP

Chloroprene
IARC 2B

Chlorothalonil
IARC 2B

para-Chloro-ortho-toluidine (and its strong acid salts)
IARC 2A, NTP

para-Chloro-ortho-toluidine Hydrochloride
NTP

Chlorozotocin
IARC 2A, NTP

Chromium compounds, hexavalent
IARC 1, NTP-1

C.I. acid red 114
IARC 2B

C.I. basic red 9
IARC 2B, NTP

C.I. direct blue 15
IARC 2B

Ciclosporin (Cylcosporine A; Ciclospirin)
IARC 1, NTP-1

Cisplatin
IARC 2A, NTP

Citrus red no. 2
IARC 2B

Clonorchis sinensis (infection with)
IARC 2A

Coal-tars
IARC 1, NTP-1

Coal-tar pitches
OSHA, IARC 1

Cobalt and cobalt compounds
IARC 2B

Coffee (urinary bladder)
IARC 2A

Coke oven emissions
OSHA*, NTP-1

Creosotes (different sources)
IARC 2A, NTP-1

para-Cresidine
IARC 2B, NTP

Cupferron
NTP

Cycasin
IARC 2B

Cyclophosphamide
IARC 1, NTP-1

Dacarbazine
IARC 2B, NTP

Danthron (1,8-dihydroxyanthraquinone)
NTP

Dantron (chrysazin;1,8-dihydroxyantraquinone)
IARC 2B, NTP

Daunomycin
IARC 2B

DDT
IARC 2B, NTP

N,N'-Diacetylbenzidine
IARC 2B

2,4-Diaminoanisole
IARC 2B

2,4-Diaminoanisole sulfate
NTP

4,4'-Diaminodiphenyl ether
IARC 2B

2,4-Diaminotoluene
IARC 2B, NTP

Dibenz[a,h]acridine
IARC 2B, NTP

Dibenz[a,j]acridine
IARC 2B, NTP

Dibenz[a,h]anthracene
IARC 2A, NTP

7H-Dibenzo[c,g]carbazole
IARC 2B, NTP

Dibenzo[a,e]pyrene
IARC 2B, NTP

Dibenzo[a,h]pyrene
IARC 2B, NTP

Dibenzo[a,i]pyrene
IARC 2B, NTP

Dibenzo[a,l]pyrene
IARC 2B, NTP

1,2-Dibromo-3-chloropropane
OSHA*, IARC 2B, NTP

1,2-Dibromoethane (EBD)
NTP

para-Dichlorobenzene
IARC 2B

ortho-Dichlorobenzene
IARC 2B

1,4-Dichlorobenzene
NTP

3,3'-Dichlorobenzidine
OSHA, IARC 2B, NTP

3,3'-Dichlorobenzidine (and its salts)
OSHA

3,3' Dichloro-4,4'diaminodiphenyl ether
IARC 2B

1,2-Dichloroethane
IARC 2B, NTP

Dichloromethane (Methylene chloride)
OSHA*, IARC 2B, NTP

1,3-Dichloropropene (technical grade)
IARC 2B, NTP

Dichlorvos
IARC 2B

Diepoxybutane
NTP

Diesel engine exhaust
IARC 2A

Diesel fuel (marine)
IARC 2B

Di(2-ethylhexyl) phthalate
IARC 2B, NTP

1,2-Diethylhydrazine
IARC 2B, NTP

Diethyl sulfate
IARC 2A, NTP

Diethylstilbestrol
IARC 1, NTP-1

Diglycidyl resorcinol ether
IARC 2B, NTP

Dihydrosafrole
IARC 2B

1,8-Dihydroxyanthraquinone
NTP

Diisopropyl sulfate
IARC 2B

3,3'-Dimethoxybenzidine (ortho-dianisidine)
IARC 2B, NTP

3,3'-Dimethoxybenzidine dihydrochloride
NTP

4-Dimethylaminoazobenzene
OSHA, NTP

para-Dimethylaminoazobenzene
IARC 2B

trans-2-[(Dimethylamino)methylimino]-5-[2-(5-nitro-2-furyl)-vinyl]-1,3,4-oxadiazole
IARC 2B

2,6-Dimethylaniline (2,6-xylidine)
IARC 2B

3,3'-Dimethylbenzidine (ortho-tolidine)
IARC 2B, NTP

Dimethylcarbamoyl chloride
IARC 2A, NTP

1,1-Dimethylhydrazine
IARC 2B, NTP

1,2-Dimethylhydrazine
IARC 2A

Dimethyl sulfate
IARC 2A, NTP

Dimethylvinyl chloride
NTP

3,7-Dinitrofluoranthrene
IARC 2B

3,9-Dinitrofluoranthrene
IARC 2B

1,6-Dinitropyrene
IARC 2B, NTP

1,8-Dinitopyrene
IARC 2B

2,4-Dinitrotoluene
IARC 2B

2,6-Dinitrotoluene
IARC 2B

1,4-Dioxane
IARC 2B, NTP

Direct black 36
NTP

Direct blue 6
NTP

Disperse blue 1
IARC 2B, NTP

Epichlorohydrin
IARC 2A, NTP

1,2-Epoxybutane
IARC 2B

Epstein-Barr virus
IARC 1

Erionite
IARC 1, NTP-1

Estrogens (conjugated)
NTP

Estrogens (not conjugated) estradiol-17 beta
NTP

Estrogens (not conjugated) estrone
NTP

Estrogens (not conjugated) ethinylestradiol
NTP

Estrogens (not conjugated) mestranol
NTP

Ethyl acrylate
IARC 2B, NTP

Ethylene dibromide
IARC 2A, NTP

Ethylene oxide
OSHA*, IARC 1, NTP

Ethyleneimine
OSHA

Ethylene thiourea
IARC 2B, NTP

Ethyl methanesulfonate
IARC 2B, NTP

N-Ethyl-N-nitrosourea
IARC 2A

Formaldehyde
OSHA*, IARC 2A, NTP

2-(2-Formylhydrazino)-4-(5-nitro-2-furyl) thiazole
IARC 2B

Fuel oils, residual
IARC 2A

Furan
IARC 2B, NTP

Fusarium moniliforme (toxins derived from)
IARC 2A

Gasoline
IARC 2B

Gasoline engine exhaust
IARC 2B

Ethylene oxide
OSHA*, IARC 1, NTP

Ethyleneimine
OSHA

Glass wool (respirable size)
IARC 2B, NTP

Glu-P-1 (2-amino-6-methyldipyrido[1,2-a:3',2'-d]imidazole)
IARC 2B

Glu-P-2 (2-aminodipyrido[1,2-a:3',2'-d]imidazole)
IARC 2B

Glycidaldehyde
IARC 2B

Glycidol
NTP

Griseofulvin
IARC 2B

HC blue no. 1
IARC 2B

Helicobacter pylori (infection with)
IARC 1

Hepatitis B virus (chronic infection with)
IARC 1

Hepatitis C virus (chronic infection with)
IARC 1

Heptachlor
IARC 2B

Hexachlorobenzene
IARC 2B, NTP

Hexachlorocyclohexanes (lindane)
IARC 2B

Hexachloroethane
IARC 2B, NTP

Hexamethylphosphoramide
IARC 2B, NTP

Human immunodeficiency virus type 1 (infection with)
IARC 1

Human immunodeficiency virus type 2 (infection with)
IARC 2B

Human papillomavirus type 16
IARC 1

Human papillomavirus type 18
IARC 1

Human papillomavirus type 31
IARC 2A

Human papillomavirus type 33
IARC 2A

Human papillomavirus (some types other than 16, 18, 31, 33)
IARC 2B

Human T-cell lymphotropic virus type I
IARC 1

Hydrazine
IARC 2B, NTP

Hydrazobenzene
NTP

Indeno[1,2,3-cd]pyrene
IARC 2B

Inorganic arsenic
OSHA*

IQ (2-Amino-3-methylimidazo[4,5-f]quinoline)
IARC 2A

Iron-dextran complex
IARC 2B, NTP

Insecticides, nonarsenical (spraying & application)
IARC 2A

Isoprene
IARC 2B

Kaposi's sarcoma herpesvirus/human herpesvirus 8
IARC 2A

Kepone (chlordecone)
IARC 2B, NTP

Lasiocarpine
IARC 2B

Lead & lead compounds, inorganic
OSHA*, IARC 2B, NTP

Lead Chromate
NTP-1

Lindane & other hexachlorocyclohexane isomers
NTP

Magenta (containing CI basic red 9)
IARC 2B

MeA-alpha-C (2-amino-3-methyl-9H-pyrido[2,3-beta]indole)
IARC 2B

MeCCNU (1,(2-Chloroethyl)-3-(4-methylhexyl)-1-nitrosourea
NTP-1

Medroxyprogesterone acetate
IARC 2B

MeIQ (2-Amino-3,4-dimethylimidazo[4,5-f]quinoline)
IARC 2B

MeIQx (2-Amino-3,8-dimethylimidazo[4,5-f]quinoxaline
IARC 2B

Melphalan
IARC 1, NTP-1

Merphalan
IARC 2B

Methoxsalen (combined with ultraviolet A therapy)
NTP-1

5-Methoxypsoralen
IARC 2A

8-Methoxypsoralen (Methoxsalen) plus ultraviolet A radiation
IARC 1

2-Methylaziridine (Propyleneimine)
IARC 2B, NTP

Methylazoxymethanol acetate
IARC 2B

Methyl chloromethyl ether
OSHA

Methyl methanesulfonate
NTP

5-Methylchrysene
IARC 2B

4,4'Methylene bis (2-chloroaniline) (MBOCA)(MOCA)
IARC 2A, NTP

4,4'Methylene bis (N,N-dimethylbenzenamine)
NTP

4,4'Methylene bis (2-methylaniline)
IARC 2B

4,4'Methylenedianiline
IARC 2B, NTP

Methylmercury compounds
IARC 2B

Methyl methanesulfonate
IARC 2A

2-Methyl-1-nitroanthraquinone (uncertain purity)
IARC 2B

N-Methyl-N'-nitro-N-nitrosoguanidine (MNNG)
IARC 2A, NTP

N-Methyl-N-nitrosourea
IARC 2A

N-Methyl-N-nitrosourethane
IARC 2B

Methylthiouracil
IARC 2B

Metronidazole
IARC 2B, NTP

Michler's ketone
NTP

Mineral oils, untreated and mildly-treated
IARC 1, NTP-1

Mirex
IARC 2B, NTP

Mitomycin C
IARC 2B

Monocrotaline
IARC 2B

MOPP (and other combined chemotherapy including alkylating agents)
IARC 1

5-(Morpholinomethyl)-3-[(5-nitrofurfurylidene) amino]-2-oxazolidinone
IARC 2B

Mustard gas (sulfur mustard)
IARC 1, NTP-1

Myleran (1,4-Butanediol dimethylsulfonate)
NTP-1

Nafenopin
IARC 2B

alpha-Naphthylamine
OSHA

beta-Naphthylamine
OSHA

2-Naphthylamine
IARC 1, NTP-1

Nickel compounds
IARC 1, NTP

Nickel, metallic
IARC 2B

Niridazole
IARC 2B

Nitrilotriacetic acid and its salts
IARC 2B, NTP

5-Nitroacenaphthene
IARC 2B

ortho-Nitroanisole (2-nitroanisole)
IARC 2B, NTP

Nitrobenzene
IARC 2B

Methylazoxymethanol and its acetate
IARC 2B

4-Nitrobiphenyl
OSHA

6-Nitrochrysene
IARC 2B, NTP

Nitrofen (Technical-grade)
IARC 2B, NTP

2-Nitrofluorene
IARC 2B

1-[(5-Nitrofurfurylidene)amino]-2-imidazolidinone
IARC 2B

N-(4-(5-Nitro-2-furyl)-2-thiazolyl)acetamide
IARC 2B

Nitrogen mustard
IARC 2A

Nitrogen mustard hydrochloride
NTP

Nitrogen mustard N-oxide
IARC 2B

2-Nitropropane
IARC 2B, NTP

1-Nitropyrene
IARC 2B, NTP

4-Nitropyrene
IARC 2B, NTP

N-Nitroso-N-ethylurea
NTP

N-Nitroso-N-methylurea
NTP

N-Nitrosodi-n-butylamine
IARC 2B, NTP

N-Nitrosodi-n-propylamine
IARC 2B, NTP

N-Nitrosodiethanolamine
IARC 2B, NTP

N-Nitrosodiethylamine
IARC 2A, NTP

N-Nitrosodimethylamine
OSHA, IARC 2A, NTP

3-(N-Nitrosomethylamino)propionitrile
IARC 2B

4-(N-Nitrosomethylamino)-1-(3-pyridyl)-1-butanone (NNK)
IARC 2B, NTP

N-Nitrosomethylethylamine
IARC 2B, NTP

N-Nitrosomethylvinylamine
IARC 2B, NTP

N-Nitrosomorpholine
IARC 2B, NTP

N'-Nitrosonornicotine
IARC 2B, NTP

N-Nitrosopiperidine
IARC 2B, NTP

N-Nitrosopyrrolidine
IARC 2B, NTP

N-Nitrososarcosine
IARC 2B, NTP

Norethisterone
NTP

Ochratoxin A
IARC 2B, NTP

Oestrogen therapy, postmenopausal
IARC 1

Oestrogen-progesterone therapy, postmenopausal
IARC 2B

Oestrogens, nonsteroidal
IARC 1

Oestrogens, steroidal
IARC 1

Oil orange SS
IARC 2B

Opisthorchis viverrini (infection with)
IARC 1

Oral contraceptives, combined
IARC 1

Oral contraceptives, sequential
IARC 1

Oxazepam
IARC 2B

4,4'-Oxydianiline
NTP

Oxymetholone
NTP

Palygorskite (attapulgite) (fibers > 5 micrometers)
IARC 2B

Panfuran S (containing dihydroxymethylfuratrizine
IARC 2B

Pentachlorophenol
IARC 2B

Phenacetin
IARC 2A, NTP

Phenazopyridine hydrochloride
IARC 2B, NTP

Phenobarbital
IARC 2B

Phenoxybenzamine hydrochloride
IARC 2B, NTP

Phenyl glycidyl ether
IARC 2B

Phenytoin
IARC 2B, NTP

PhIP (2-Amino-1-methyl-6-phenylimidazo[4,5-beta]pyridine)
IARC 2B

Piperazine estrone sulfate (as conjugated estrogen)
NTP-1

Polybrominated biphenyls
IARC 2B, NTP

Polychlorinated biphenyls
IARC 2A, NTP

Polychlorinated camphenes
IARC 2A

Polychlorophenols and their sodium salts (mixed exposures)
IARC 2B

Polycyclic aromatic hydrocarbons, 15 Listings
NTP

Benz (a) anthracene
IARC 2A, NTP

Benzo (b) fluoranthene
IARC 2B, NTP

Benzo (j) fluoranthene
IARC 2B, NTP

Benzo (k) fluoranthene
IARC 2B, NTP

Benzo (a) pyrene
IARC 2A, NTP

Dibenz (a,h) acridine
IARC 2B, NTP

Dibenz (a,j) acridine
IARC 2B, NTP

Dibenz (a,h) anthracene
IARC 2A, NTP

7H-Dibenzo (c,g) carbazole
IARC 2B, NTP

Dibenzo (a,e) pyrene
IARC 2B, NTP

Dibenzo (a,h) pyrene
IARC 2B, NTP

Dibenzo (a,i) pyrene
IARC 2B, NTP

Dibenzo (a,l) pyrene
IARC 2B, NTP

Indeno (1,2,3-cd) pyrene
IARC 2B, NTP

5-Methylchrysene
IARC 2B, NTP

Ponceau MX
IARC 2B

Ponceau 3R
IARC 2B

Potassium bromate
IARC 2B

Procarbazine hydrochloride
IARC 2A, NTP

Progesterone
IARC 2B, NTP

Progestins
IARC 2B

1,3-Propane sultone
IARC 2B, NTP

beta-Propiolactone
OSHA, IARC 2B, NTP

Propylene oxide
IARC 2B, NTP

Propylthiouracil
IARC 2B, NTP

Radon
IARC 1, NTP-1

Reserpine
NTP

Rockwool
IARC 2B

Saccharin
NTP

Safrole
IARC 2B, NTP

Schistosoma haematobium (infection with)
IARC 1

Schistosoma japonicum (infection with)
IARC 2B

Selenium sulfide
NTP

Shale-oils
IARC 1

Silica, crystalline (respirable size)
NTP

Cristobalite
IARC 1, NTP

Quartz
IARC 1, NTP

Tridymite
NTP

Slagwool
IARC 2B

Sodium equilin sulfate (as conjugated estrogen)
NTP-1

Sodium estrone sulfate (as conjugated estrogen)
NTP-1

Sodium ortho-phenylphenate
IARC 2B

Soots, tars and mineral oils
IARC 1, NTP

Sterigmatocystin
IARC 2B

Streptozotocin
IARC 2B, NTP

Strong inorganic acid mists containing sulfuric acid
IARC 1

Strontium chromate
NTP-1

Styrene
IARC 2B

Styrene-7,8-oxide
IARC 2A

Sulfallate
IARC 2B, NTP

Talc containing asbestiform fibers
IARC 1

Tamoxifen
IARC 1

Tars
NTP-1

2,3,7,8-Tetrachlorodibenzo-para-dioxin (TCDD)
IARC 1, NTP

Tetrachloroethylene (Perchloroethylene)
IARC 2A, NTP

Tetrafluoroethylene
IARC 2B

Tetranitromethane
IARC 2B, NTP

Thioacetimide
IARC 2B, NTP

4,4'-Thiodianiline
IARC 2B

Thiotepa (Tris(1-aziridinyl)phosphine sulfide)
IARC 1, NTP-1

Thiourea
IARC 2B, NTP

Thorium Dioxide
NTP-1

Tobacco products, smokeless
IARC 1

Tobacco smoke
IARC 1

Toluene diisocyanates
IARC 2B, NTP

ortho-Toluidine
IARC 2B, NTP

Toxaphene (polychlorinated camphenes)
IARC 2B, NTP

Treosulfan
IARC 1

Trichloroethylene
IARC 2A

Trichlormethine (trimustine hydrochloride)
IARC 2B

2,4,6-Trichlorophenol
IARC 2B, NTP

1,2,3-Trichloropropane
IARC 2A, NTP

Tris(1-aziridinyl)phosphine sulfide(thiotepa)
IARC 1, NTP-1

Tris (2,3-dibromopropyl)phosphate
IARC 2A, NTP

Trp-P-1 (3-amino-1,4-dimethyl-5H-pyrido[4,3-b]indole)
IARC 2B

Trp-P-2 (3-amino-1-methyl-5H-pyrido[4,3-b]indole)
IARC 2B

Trypan blue
IARC 2B

Uracil mustard
IARC 2B

Urethane
IARC 2B, NTP

Vinyl acetate
IARC 2B

Vinyl bromide
IARC 2A

Vinyl chloride
OSHA*, IARC 1, NTP-1

4-Vinylcyclohexene
IARC 2B

4-Vinyl-1-cyclohexene diepoxide
IARC 2B, NTP

Vinyl fluoride
IARC 2A

Welding fumes
IARC 2B

Wood Dust
IARC I

Zinc chromate
NTP-1

OSHA* indicates substances for which OSHA has promulgated expanded health standards that govern health concerns in addition to carcinogenicity

Source: HAZARD Database. Chemical Teratogens, Carcinogens, Mutagens. List of Carcinogens. Accessible at www.iephb.nw.ru/~spirov/hazard/carcinogen_lst.html.

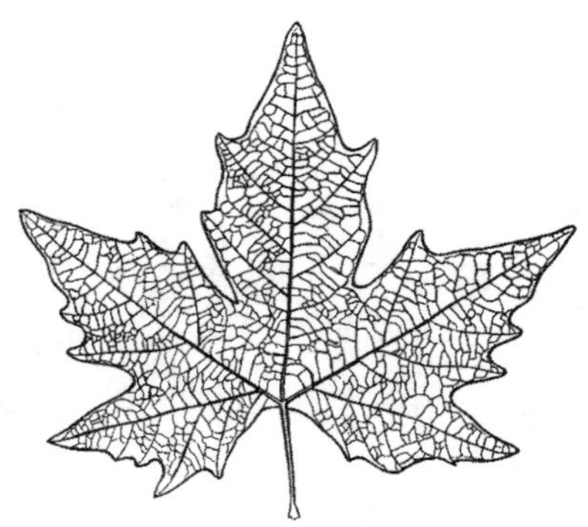

APPENDIX C

CARCINOGENS ACCORDING TO CALIFORNIA PROPOSITION 65

Proposition 65, the Safe Drinking Water and Toxic Enforcement Act of 1986, requires the governor of California to publish annually a list of chemicals known in the state to cause cancer and birth defects. The list below includes only those chemicals associated with a risk of cancer.

Chemical

A-alpha-C (2-Amino-9H-pyrido[2,3-b]indole)

Acetaldehyde

Acetamide

Acetochlor

2-Acetylaminofluorene

Acifluorfen

Acrylamide

Acrylonitrile

Actinomycin D

Adriamycin (Doxorubicin hydrochloride)

AF-2;[2-(2-furyl)-3-(5-nitro-2-furyl)]acrylamide

Aflatoxins

Alachlor

Alcoholic beverages, when associated with alcohol abuse

Aldrin

2-Aminoanthraquinone

p-Aminoazobenzene

o-Aminoazotoluene

4-Aminobiphenyl (4-amino-diphenyl)

1-Amino-2,4-dibromoanthraquinone

3-Amino-9-ethylcarbazole hydrochloride

2-Aminofluorene

1-Amino-2-methylanthraquinone

2-Amino-5-(5-nitro-2-furyl)-1,3,4-thiadiazole

4-Amino-2-nitrophenol

Amitrole

Anabolic steroids

Analgesic mixtures containing Phenacetin

Aniline

Aniline hydrochloride

o-Anisidine

o-Anisidine hydrochloride

Antimony oxide (Antimony trioxide)

Aramite

Areca nut

Aristolochic acids

Arsenic (inorganic arsenic compounds)

Asbestos

Auramine

Azacitidine

Azaserine

Azathioprine

Azobenzene

Benz[a]anthracene

Benzene

Benzidine [and its salts]

Benzidine-based dyes

Benzo[b]fluoranthene

Benzo[j]fluoranthene

Benzo[k]fluoranthene

Benzofuran

Benzo[a]pyrene

Benzotrichloride

Benzyl chloride

Benzyl violet 4B

Beryllium and beryllium compounds

Betel quid with tobacco

Betel quid without tobacco

2,2-Bis(bromomethyl)-1,3-propanediol

Bis(2-chloroethyl)ether

N,N-Bis(2-chloroethyl)-2-naphthylamine (Chlornapazine)

Bischloroethyl nitrosourea (BCNU) (Carmustine)

Bis(chloromethyl)ether

Bis(2-chloro-1-methylethyl)ether, technical grade

Bitumens, extracts of steam-refined and air refined

Bracken fern

Bromacil lithium salt

Bromate

Bromodichloromethane

Bromoethane

Bromoform

2-Bromopropane

1,3-Butadiene

1,4-Butanediol dimethanesulfonate (Busulfan)

Butylated hydroxyanisole

beta-Butyrolactone

Cacodylic acid

Cadmium and cadmium compounds

Caffeic acid

Captafol

Captan

Carbazole

Carbon black (airborne, unbound particles of respirable size)

Carbon tetrachloride

Carbon-black extracts

N-Carboxymethyl-N-nitrosourea

Catechol

Ceramic fibers (airborne particles of respirable size)

Certain combined chemotherapy for lymphomas

Chlorambucil

Chloramphenicol

Chlordane

Chlordecone (Kepone)

Chlordimeform

Chlorendic acid

Chlorinated paraffins (Average chain length, C12;approximately 60 percent chlorine by weight)

p-Chloroaniline

p-Chloroaniline hydrochloride

Chloroethane (Ethyl chloride)

1-(2-Chloroethyl)-3-cyclohexyl-1-nitrosourea (CCNU) (Lomustine)

1-(2-Chloroethyl)-3-(4-methylcyclohexyl)-1-nitrosourea (Methyl-CCNU)

Chloroform

Chloromethyl methyl ether (technical grade)

3-Chloro-2-methylpropene

1-Chloro-4-nitrobenzene

4-Chloro-*o*-phenylenediamine

Chloroprene

Chlorothalonil

p-Chloro-*o*-toluidine

p-Chloro-*o*-toluidine, strong acid salts of

5-Chloro-*o*-toluidine and its strong acid salts

Chlorotrianisene

Chlorozotocin

Chromium (hexavalent compounds)

Chrysene

C.I. Acid Red 114

C.I. Basic Red 9 monohydrochloride

C.I. Direct Blue 15

C.I. Direct Blue 218

C.I. Solvent Yellow 14

Ciclosporin (Cyclosporin A; Cyclosporine)

Cidofovir

Cinnamyl anthranilate

Cisplatin

Citrus Red No. 2

Clofibrate

Cobalt metal powder

Cobalt [II] oxide

Cobalt sulfate

Cobalt sulfate heptahydrate

Coke oven emissions

Conjugated estrogens

Creosotes

p-Cresidine
Cupferron
Cycasin
Cyclophosphamide (anhydrous)
Cyclophosphamide (hydrated)
Cytembena
D&C Orange No. 17
D&C Red No. 8
D&C Red No. 9
D&C Red No. 19
Dacarbazine
Daminozide
Dantron (Chrysazin; 1,8-Dihydroxyanthraquinone)
Daunomycin
DDD (Dichlorodiphenyl-dichloroethane)
DDE (Dichlorodiphenyl-dichloroethylene)
DDT (Dichlorodiphenyl-trichloroethane)
DDVP (Dichlorvos)
N,N'-Diacetylbenzidine
2,4-Diaminoanisole
2,4-Diaminoanisole sulfate
4,4'-Diaminodiphenyl ether (4,4'-Oxydianiline)
2,4-Diaminotoluene
Diaminotoluene (mixed)
Diazoaminobenzene
Dibenz[a,h]acridine
Dibenz[a,j]acridine
Dibenz[a,h]anthracene
7H-Dibenzo[c,g]carbazole
Dibenzo[a,e]pyrene
Dibenzo[a,h]pyrene
Dibenzo[a,i]pyrene
Dibenzo[a,l]pyrene
1,2-Dibromo-3-chloropropane (DBCP)
1,2-Dibromo-3-chloropropane (DBCP)
2,3-Dibromo-1-propanol
Dichloroacetic acid
p-Dichlorobenzene
3,3'-Dichlorobenzidine
3,3'-Dichlorobenzidine dihydrochloride
1,4-Dichloro-2-butene
3,3'-Dichloro-4,4'-diamino-diphenyl ether
1,1-Dichloroethane
Dichloromethane (Methylene chloride)
1,2-Dichloropropane
1,3-Dichloropropene
Dieldrin
Dienestrol
Diepoxybutane
Diesel engine exhaust
Di(2-ethylhexyl)phthalate
1,2-Diethylhydrazine
Diethylstilbestrol (DES)
Diethyl sulfate
Diglycidyl resorcinol ether (DGRE)
Dihydrosafrole
Diisopropyl sulfate
3,3'-Dimethoxybenzidine (*o*-Dianisidine)
3,3'-Dimethoxybenzidine dihydrochloride

3,3'-Dimethoxybenzidine-based dyes metabolized to 3,3'-dimethoxybenzidine

4-Dimethylaminoazobenzene

trans-2-[(Dimethylamino)methylimino]-5-[2-(5-nitro-2-furyl)vinyl]-1,3,4-oxadiazole

7,12-Dimethylbenz(a)anthracene

3,3'-Dimethylbenzidine (ortho-Tolidine)

3,3'-Dimethylbenzidine dihydrochloride

3,3'-Dimethylbenzidine-based dyes metabolized to 3,3'-dimethylbenzidine

Dimethylcarbamoyl chloride

1,1-Dimethylhydrazine (UDMH)

1,2-Dimethylhydrazine

Dimethyl sulfate

Dimethylvinylchloride

m-Dinitrobenzene

o-Dinitrobenzene

p-Dinitrobenzene

3,7-Dinitrofluoranthene

3,9-Dinitrofluoranthene

1,6-Dinitropyrene

1,8-Dinitropyrene

Dinitrotoluene mixture, 2,4-/2,6-

2,4-Dinitrotoluene

2,6-Dinitrotoluene

1,4-Dioxane

Diphenylhydantoin (Phenytoin)

Diphenylhydantoin (Phenytoin), sodium salt

Di-*n*-propyl isocinchomeronate (MGK Repellent 326)

Direct Black 38 (technical grade)

Direct Blue 6 (technical grade)

Direct Brown 95 (technical grade)

Disperse Blue 1

Diuron

Epichlorohydrin

Erionite

Estradiol 17B

Estragole

Estrogens, steroidal

Estrone

Estropipate

Ethinylestradiol

Ethoprop

Ethyl acrylate

Ethylbenzene

Ethyl-4,4'-dichlorobenzilate

Ethylene dibromide

Ethylene dichloride (1,2-Dichloroethane)

Ethyleneimine

Ethylene oxide

Ethylene oxide

Ethylene thiourea

Ethyl methanesulfonate

Fenoxycarb

Folpet

Formaldehyde (gas)

2-(2-Formylhydrazino)-4-(5-nitro-2-furyl)thiazole

Fumonisin B_1

Furan

Furazolidone

Furmecyclox

Fusarin C

Ganciclovir sodium

Gasoline engine exhaust (condensates/extracts)

Gemfibrozil

Glass wool fibers (airborne particles of respirable size)

Glu-P-1 (2-Amino-6-methyldipyrido[1,2-a:3',2'-d]imidazole)

Glu-P-2 (2-Aminodipyrido[1,2-a:3',2'-d]imidazole)

Glycidaldehyde

Glycidol

Griseofulvin

Gyromitrin (Acetaldehyde methylformylhydrazone)

HC Blue 1

Heptachlor

Heptachlor epoxide

Herbal remedies containing plant species of the genus Aristolochia

Hexachlorobenzene

Hexachlorocyclohexane (technical grade)

Hexachlorodibenzodioxin

Hexachloroethane

2,4-Hexadienal (89% trans, trans isomer; 11% cis, trans isomer)

Hexamethylphosphoramide

Hydrazine

Hydrazine sulfate

Hydrazobenzene (1,2-Diphenylhydrazine)

1-Hydroxyanthraquinone

Indeno [1,2,3-cd]pyrene

Indium phosphide

IQ (2-Amino-3-methylimidazo[4,5-f] quinoline)

Iprodione

Iron dextran complex

Isobutyl nitrite

Isoprene

Isosafrole

Isoxaflutole

Lactofen

Lasiocarpine

Lead and lead compounds

Lead acetate

Lead phosphate

Lead subacetate

Lindane and other hexachlorocyclohexane isomers

Medroxyprogesterone acetate

MeIQ (2-Amino-3,4-dimethylimidazo[4,5-f]quinoline)

MeIQx (2-Amino-3,8-dimethylimidazo[4,5-f]quinoxaline)

Melphalan

Merphalan

Mestranol

Metham sodium

5-Methoxypsoralen with ultraviolet A therapy

8-Methoxypsoralen with ultraviolet A therapy

2-Methylaziridine (Propyleneimine)

Methylazoxymethanol

Methylazoxymethanol acetate

Methyl carbamate

3-Methylcholanthrene

5-Methylchrysene

4,4'-Methylene bis(2-chloroaniline)

4,4'-Methylene bis(N,N-dimethyl)benzenamine

4,4'-Methylene bis(2-methylaniline)

4,4'-Methylenedianiline

4,4'-Methylenedianiline dihydrochloride

Methyleugenol

Methylhydrazine and its salts

Methyl iodide

Methylmercury compounds

Methyl methanesulfonate

2-Methyl-1-nitroanthraquinone (of uncertain purity)

N-Methyl-N'-nitro-N-nitrosoguanidine

N-Methylolacrylamide

Methylthiouracil

Metiram

Metronidazole

Michler's ketone

Mirex

Mitomycin C

Monocrotaline

5-(Morpholinomethyl)-3-[(5-nitrofurfurylidene)-amino]-2-oxazolidinone

Mustard Gas

MX (3-chloro-4-dichloromethyl-5-hydroxy-2(5H)-furanone)

Nafenopin

Nalidixic acid

Naphthalene

1-Naphthylamine

2-Naphthylamine

Nickel (Metallic)

Nickel acetate

Nickel carbonate

Nickel carbonyl

Nickel compounds

Nickel hydroxide

Nickelocene

Nickel oxide

Nickel refinery dust from the pyrometallurgical process

Nickel subsulfide

Niridazole

Nitrapyrin

Nitrilotriacetic acid

Nitrilotriacetic acid, trisodium salt monohydrate

5-Nitroacenaphthene

5-Nitro-*o*-anisidine

o-Nitroanisole

Nitrobenzene

4-Nitrobiphenyl

6-Nitrochrysene

Nitrofen (technical grade)

2-Nitrofluorene

Nitrofurantoin

Nitrofurazone

1-[(5-Nitrofurfurylidene)-amino]-2-imidazolidinone

N-[4-(5-Nitro-2-furyl)-2-thiazolyl]acetamide

Nitrogen mustard (Mechlorethamine)

Nitrogen mustard hydrochloride (Mechlorethamine hydrochloride)

Nitrogen mustard N-oxide

Nitrogen mustard N-oxide hydrochloride

Nitromethane

2-Nitropropane

1-Nitropyrene

4-Nitropyrene

N-Nitrosodi-*n*-butylamine

N-Nitrosodiethanolamine

N-Nitrosodiethylamine

N-Nitrosodimethylamine

p-Nitrosodiphenylamine

N-Nitrosodiphenylamine

N-Nitrosodi-*n*-propylamine

N-Nitroso-N-ethylurea

3-(N-Nitrosomethylamino) propionitrile

4-(N-Nitrosomethylamino)-1-(3-pyridyl)1-butanone

N-Nitrosomethylethylamine

N-Nitroso-N-methylurea

N-Nitroso-N-methylurethane

N-Nitrosomethylvinylamine

N-Nitrosomorpholine

N-Nitrosonornicotine

N-Nitrosopiperidine

N-Nitrosopyrrolidine

N-Nitrososarcosine

o-Nitrotoluene

Norethisterone (Norethindrone)

Norethynodrel

Ochratoxin A

Oil Orange SS

Oral contraceptives, combined

Oral contraceptives, sequential

Oxadiazon

Oxazepam

Oxymetholone

Oxythioquinox

Palygorskite fibers (> 5μm in length)

Panfuran S

Pentachlorophenol

Phenacetin

Phenazopyridine

Phenazopyridine hydrochloride

Phenesterin

Phenobarbital

Phenolphthalein

Phenoxybenzamine

Phenoxybenzamine hydrochloride

o-Phenylenediamine and its salts

Phenyl glycidyl ether

Phenylhydrazine and its salts

o-Phenylphenate, sodium

o-Phenylphenol

PhiP(2-Amino-1-methyl-6-phenylimidazol[4,5-b]pyridine)

Polybrominated biphenyls

Polychlorinated biphenyls

Polychlorinated biphenyls (containing 60 or more percent percent chlorine by molecular weight)

Polychlorinated dibenzo-*p*-dioxins

Polychlorinated dibenzofurans

Polygeenan

Ponceau MX

Ponceau 3R

Potassium bromate

Primidone

Procarbazine

Procarbazine hydrochloride

Procymidone

Progesterone

Pronamide

Propachlor

1,3-Propane sultone

Propargite

beta-Propiolactone

Propylene glycol mono-*t*-butyl ether

Propylene oxide

Propylthiouracil

Pyridine

Quinoline and its strong acid salts

Radionuclides

Reserpine

Residual (heavy) fuel oils

Riddelliine

Safrole

Salicylazosulfapyridine

Selenium sulfide

Shale-oils

Silica, crystalline (airborne particles of respirable size)

Soots, tars, and mineral oils (untreated and mildly treated oils and used engine oils)

Spironolactone

Stanozolol

Sterigmatocystin

Streptozotocin (streptozocin)

Strong inorganic acid mists containing sulfuric acid

Styrene oxide

Sulfallate

Talc containing asbestiform fibers

Tamoxifen and its salts

Terrazole

Testosterone and its esters

2,3,7,8-Tetrachlorodibenzo-*p*-dioxin (TCDD)

1,1,2,2-Tetrachloroethane

Tetrachloroethylene (Perchloroethylene)

p-a,a,a-Tetrachlorotoluene

Tetrafluoroethylene

Tetranitromethane

Thioacetamide

4,4'-Thiodianiline

Thiodicarb

Thiouracil

Thiourea

Thorium dioxide

Tobacco, oral use of smokeless products

Tobacco smoke

Toluene diisocyanate

o-Toluidine

o-Toluidine hydrochloride

Toxaphene (Polychlorinated camphenes)

Treosulfan

Trichlormethine (Trimustine hydrochloride)

Trichloroethylene

2,4,6-Trichlorophenol

1,2,3-Trichloropropane

2,4,5-Trimethylaniline and its strong acid salts

Trimethyl phosphate

Triphenyltin hydroxide

Tris(aziridinyl)-*p*-benzoquinone (Triaziquone)

Tris(1-aziridinyl)phosphine sulfide (Thiotepa)

Tris(2-chloroethyl) phosphate

Tris(2,3-dibromopropyl)phosphate

Trp-P-1 (Tryptophan-P-1)

Trp-P-2 (Tryptophan-P-2)

Trypan blue (commercial grade)

Unleaded gasoline (wholly vaporized)

Uracil mustard

Urethane (Ethyl carbamate)

Vanadium pentoxide (orthorhombic crystalline form)

Vinclozolin

Vinyl bromide

Vinyl chloride

4-Vinylcyclohexene

4-Vinyl-1-cyclohexene diepoxide (Vinyl cyclohexenedioxide)

Vinyl fluoride

Vinyl trichloride (1,1,2-Trichloroethane)

2,6-Xylidine (2,6-Dimethylaniline)

Zileuton

OSHA* indicates substances for which OSHA has promulgated expanded health standards that govern health concerns in addition to carcinogenicity

Source: State of California. Environmental Protection Agency. Office of Environmental Health Hazard Assessment. Safe Drinking Water and Toxic Enforcement Act of 1986. Chemicals Known to the State to Cause Cancer or Reproductive Toxicity. June 9, 2006. Accessed at www.oehha.ca.gov/prop65/prop65_list/files/060906P65single.pdf.

References

Acrylamide

Acrylamide and Proposition 65. OEHHA – Office of Environmental Health Hazard Assessment. 2005. Accessed 01/26/06 at www.oehha.ca.gov/prop65/acrylamideqa.html.

FDA data on Acrylamide concentration in Foods. US FDA 2004. Accessed 07/05/06 at www.oehha.ca.gov/prop65/acrylamideintakefdaappendix.pdf.

Michels, KB, et al. 2005. Preschool diet and risk of breast cancer. *International Journal of Cancer.* 118:749-754.

Office of the Attorney General. State of California. Department of Justice. Attorney General Lockyer files suit to require common warnings about cancer-causing chemical in Potato chips and French fries. Action against nine firms warnings on acrylamide required by proposition 65. Accessed 07/05/06 at http://ag.ca.gov/newsalerts/release.php?id=1207.

Summary of acrylamide intake estimates. OEEHA. Accessed 07/05/06 at www.oehha.ca.gov/prop65/acrylamideintaketable2.doc

Tareke, E. et al. 2002. Analysis of acrylamide, a carcinogen formed in heated food stuffs. *Journal of Agricultural and Food Chemistry.* 50:4998-5006.

Alcohol

Boffetta, P. et al. 2006. The burden of cancer attributable to alcohol drinking. *International Journal of Cancer.* 119:884-887.

Hilakivi-Clarke, L. et al. 2004. In utero alcohol exposure increases mammary tumorigenesis in rats. *British Journal of Cancer.* 90:2225-2241.

Horn-Ross, P. 2004. Patterns of Alcohol Consumption and Breast Cancer Risk in the California Teachers Study Cohort. *Cancer Epidemiology Biomarkers and Prevention.* 13:405-411.

Anabolic steroids

Buckley, W. et al. 1998. Estimated Prevalence of Anabolic Steroid use among Male High School Seniors. *The Journal of the American Medical Association.* 260:3446-3450.

Antibiotics

Velicer, C. et al. 2004. Antibiotics Use in the Relation to Breast Cancer. *The Journal of the American Medical Association.* 291:827-835.

Antioxidant supplements

Blot, W. et al. 1994. Nutrition Intervention Trials in Linixan, China: Supplementation with Specific Vitamin/Mineral Combinations, Cancer Incidence, and Disease. Specific mortality in the General Population. *Journal of the National Cancer Institute.* 85:1483-1491.

Meyer, F. et al. 2005. Antioxidant vitamin and mineral supplementation and prostate cancer prevention in the SU.VI.MAX trial. *International Journal of Cancer.* 116:182-186.

Omenn, G.S. et al. 1994. The beta-carotene and retinol efficacy trial (CARET) for chemoprevention of lung cancer in high risk populations: Smokers and asbestos-exposed workers. *Cancer Research.* 54:2038S-2043S.

The Alpha-Tocopherol, Beta Carotene Cancer Prevention Study Group. 1994. The effects of vitamin E and beta carotene on the incidence of lung cancer and other cancers in male smokers. *The New England Journal of Medicine.* 330:1029-1035.

Apples

Xing, N. et al. 2001. Quercetin inhibits the expression and function of the androgen receptor in LNCaP prostate cancer cells. *Carcinogenesis.* 22:409-414,

Marchand, L. et al. 2000. Intake of flavonoids and lung cancer. *Journal of the National Cancer Institute.* 92:154-160.

Gallus, S. et al. 2005. Does an apple a day keep the oncologist away? *Annals of Oncology.* 16:1841-1844.

Tsao, R. et al. 2005. Which Polyphenolic Compounds Contribute to the Total Antioxidant activities of Apples? *Journal of Agricultural and Food Chemistry.* 53:4989-4995.

Arsenic/playground equipment

Cancellation of Residential uses of CCA-treated wood. Questions and answers. March 2003. United States Environmental Protection Agency. Accessed 04/02/06 at www.epa.gov/pesticides/factsheets/chemical/1file.htm

A Probabilistic risk assessment for children who contact CCA treated play sets and decks. Nov 2003. United States Environmental Protection Agency. Accessed 04/02/06 at www.epa/gov/scipoly/sap

Petition to the United States Consumer Product Safety Commission to Ban Arsenic Treated Wood in Playground Equipment and Review the Safety of Arsenic Treated Wood for General Use. May 2001. Environmental Working Group. Accessed 04/02/06 at www.Ewg.org/reports/poisonedplaygrounds/petition.pdf.

B-carotene, smokers

Albanes, D. 1996. a-Tocopherol and b-Carotene Supplements and Lung Cancer Incidence in the alpha-Tocopherol, beta-Carotene Cancer Prevention Study: Effects of Base-line Characteristics and Study Compliance. *Journal of the National Cancer Institute.* 88:1560-1570.

Beans

Adebamowo, C. et al. 2005. Dietary flavonols and flavonol-rich foods intake and risk of breast cancer. *International Journal of Cancer.* 114; 628-633.

Gurfinkel, D.M., and A.V. Rao. 2003. Soya saponins: The relationship Between Chemical Structure and Colon Anticarcinogenic Activity. *Nutrition and Cancer.* 47: 24-33.

Koratka, R., and A.V. Rao. 1997. Effect of soya bean saponins on azoxymethatne-induced preneoplastic lesions in the colon of mice. *Nutrition and Cancer.* 27; 206-209.

Bovine growth hormone, Insulin-like growth factor (IGF-1)

Chan, J. et al. 1998. Plasma Insulin-like growth Factor 1 and Prostate Cancer Risk: A Prospective Study. *Science.* 279:563-566.

Cleveland, R. et al. 2006. IGF1 CA repeat polymorphisms, lifestyle factors and breast cancer risk in the Long Island Breast Cancer Study Project. *Carcinogenesis.* 27:758-765.

Daughaday, W., and D.Barbano. 1990. Bovine somatotropin supplementation of dairy cows – Is the milk safe? *The Journal of the American Medical Association.* 264:1003-1005.

Hankinson, S. et al. 1998. Circulating concentrations of insulin-like growth factor 1 and risk of breast cancer. *Lancet.* 351:1393-1396.

Holly, J. 1998. Insulin-like growth factor-1 and new opportunities for cancer prevention. *Lancet.* 351:1373-1375.

IGF-1, Milk and Cancer. *Consumer Reports.* 2000. Accessed 06/24/06 at www.igf-1and-milk.com/igf-1-consumer-reports.htm.

Kodoma, Y. et al. 2002. The mouse rasH2/BHT model as an in vivo rapid assay for lung carcinogens. *Japanese Journal of Cancer Research.* 93:861-866.

NIH technology assessment conference statement on bovine somatotropin. 1991. *The Journal of the American Medical Association.* 1423-1425.

Breastfeeding

Andrieu, N. et al. 2006. Pregnancies, Breast-Feeding, and Breast Cancer Risk in the International BRCA1/2 Carrier Cohort Study (IBCCS). *Journal of the National Cancer Institute.* 98:535-544.

Bener, A. et al. 2001. Longer breastfeeding and protection against chilhood leukaemia and lymphomas. *European Journal of Cancer.* 37:234-238.

Davis, MK. 1998. Review of the evidence for an association between infant breastfeeding and childhood cancer. *International Journal of Cancer Supplement.* 11:29-33.

Kwan, M.L. et al. 2004. Breast feeding and the risk of childhood leukemia: A meta-analysis. *Public Health Reports.* 119:521-535.

Rosenblatt, K.A. and D.B. Thomas. 1993. Lactation and the risk of epithelial ovarian cancer. WHO Collaborative Study of Neoplasia and Steroid Contraceptives. *International Journal of Epidemiology.* 22:192-197.

Shu, X.O. et al. 1999. Breast-feeding and risk of childhood acute leukemia. *Journal of the National Cancer Institute.* 91:1765-1772.

Smulevich, V et al. 1999. Parental Occupation and other factors and cancer risk in children: I. Study Methodology and non-occupational factors. *International Journal of Cancer.* 83:712-717.

Breast implants

Brinton, L. et al. 2000. Breast Cancer Following Augmentation Mammoplasty (United States). *Cancer Causes and Control.* 11:819-827.

Brinton, L. et al. 2000. Characteristics of a Population of Women with Breast implants compared with women seeking other types of plastic surgery. *Plastic and Reconstructive Surgery.* 105:919-927.

Segal, M. November 1995. A status report on Breast implant Safety. United States Food and Drug Administration. *FDA Consumer Magazine.* Accessed 03/26/06 at www.fdc.gov/FDAC/features/995_implants.html.

Calcium

Baron, J et al. 1999. Calcium Supplements for the Prevention of Colorectal Adenomas. *The New England Journal of Medicine.* 340:101-107.

Jackson, R. et al. 2006. Calcium plus Vitamin D Supplementation and the Risk of Fractures. *The The New England Journal of Medicine.* 354:669-683.

Wactawski-Wende, J. et al. 2006. Calcium plus Vitamin D Supplementation and the Risk of Colorectal Cancer. *The New England Journal of Medicine.* 354:684-696.

Cancer Epidemiology

American Cancer Society. Cancer Facts and Figures 2006. Accessed 05/26/06 at www.cancer.org/downloads/STT/CPED2006PWSecured.pdf

CIA. The World Factbook 2006. Rank Order – Life Expectancy at Birth. Accessed 08/15/06 at www.cia.gov/cia/publications/factbook/rankorder/2102rank.html.

CDC National Center for Health Statistics. Table 29. Age-adjusted death rates for selected causes of death, according to sex, race, and Hispanic origin. United States, selected years 1950-2003. (updated 2006) Accessed 06/24/06 at http://www.cdc.gov/nchs/data/hus/hus05.pdf#029

Global cancer rates could increase by 50% to 15 million by 2020. World Health Organization. Accessed 04/10/2006 at www.who.intl/mediacentre/news/releases/2003/rr27/en/index.html.

Oliveria, S.A., P.J. Christos, and M. Berwick. 1997. The Role of Epidemiology in Cancer Prevention. *The Society for Experimental Biology and Medicine.* 216:142-150.

Ropeik, D. and G. Gray. "Risk: A Practical Guide for Deciding What's Really Safe and What's Really Dangerous in the World Around You." 2002. New York: Houghton Mifflin Company.

Scottenfeld, D., and J. Beebe-Dimmer. 2006. Chronic Inflammation: A Common and Important Factor in the Pathogenesis of Neoplasia. *CA. A Cancer Journal for Clinicians.* 56:69-83.

World Health Organization. Accessed 03/13/06 at www.who.int/mediacentre/new/releases/2003/pr27/en/.

Cancer screening

Schwartz, L. et al. 2004. Enthusiasm for Screening in the United States. *The Journal of the American Medical Association.* 291:71-78.

Carbonated beverages

Mayne, S. et al. 2006. Carbonated soft drink consumption and risk of esophageal adenocarcinoma. *Journal of the National Cancer Institute.* 98:72-75.

Carrots

Kobaek-Larsen, M. et al. 2005. Inhibitory effects of feeding with carrots or falcarinol on development of azoxymethano-induced colo preneoplastic lesions in rats. *Journal of Agricultural and Food Chemistry.* 53: 1823-1827.

Talcott, S.T., et al. 2000. Antioxidant changes and sensory properties of carrot puree processed with and without periderm tissue. *Journal of Agricultural and Food Chemistry.* 48: 1315-1321.

Cats

Malone, GE et al. 1983. A review of evidence that the feline leukemia virus might be causative in childhood ALL. *Cancer Treatment Research.* 17:45-65.

Cell phones

Cell phone facts. Consumer information on Wireless Phones. FDA. Accessed 03/30/06 at www.fda.gov/cellphones/wireless.html#2.

Lonn, S. et al. 2004. Mobile phone use and the risk of acoustic neuroma. *Epidemiology.* 15:653-659.

Cocoa

Lee, K. Won et al. 2003. Cocoa has more phenolic phytochemicals and a higher antioxidant capacity than teas and red wine. *Journal of Agricultural and Food Chemistry.* 51:7292-7295.

Coffee

Michels, K.B. et al. 2005. Coffee, tea, and caffeine consumption and incidence of colon and rectal cancer. *Journal of the National Cancer Institute.* 4:282-292.

Inoue, M. et al. 2005. Influence of Coffee Drinking on Subsequent Risk of Hepatocellular Carcinoma: A Prospective Study in Japan. *Journal of the National Cancer Institute.* 97:293-300.

Villanueva, C.M. et al. 2006. Total and specific fluid consumption as determinants of bladder cancer risk. *International Journal of Cancer.* 118:2040-2047.

Colon polyps

Bond, J.H. 2000. Diagnosis, treatment, and surveillance for patients with colorectal polyps. *The American Journal of Gastroenterology.* 95:3053-3063.

Walsh, J., and J.Terdiman. 2003. Colorectal Cancer Screening: Scientific Review. *The Journal of the American Medical Association.* 289:1288-1296.

Conjugated linoleic acid

Aro, A. et al. 2000. Inverse association between dietary and serum conjugated linoleic acid and risk of breast cancer in postmenopausal women. *Nutrition and Cancer.* 38:151-157.

Degner, S.C. et al. 2006. Conjugated linoleic acid attenuates cyclooxygenase-2 transcriptional activity via an anti-AP-1 mechanism in MCF-7 breast cancer cells. *Journal of Nutrition.* 136:421-427.

De La Torre, A. et al. 2006. Beef conjugated linoleic acid isomers reduce human cancer cell growth even when associated with other beef fatty acids. *British Journal of Nutrition.* 95:346-352.

Dhiman, T.R., S.H. Nam, and A.L. Ure. 2005. Factors affecting conjugated linoleic acid content in milk and meat. *Critical Reviews in Food Science and Nutrition.* 46:463-482.

French, P. et al. 2000. Fatty acid composition, including conjugated linoleic acid, of intramuscular fat from steers offered grazed grass, grass silage, or concentrate-based diets. *Journal of Animal Science.* 78:2849-2855.

Lee, S.H. et al. 2006. Conjugated linoleic acid stimulates an anti-tumorigenic protein NAG-1 in an isomer specific manner. *Carcinogenesis.* 27:972-981.

McCann, S.E. et al. 2004. Dietary intake of conjugated linoleic acids and risk of premenopausal and postmenopausal breast cancer, Western New York Exposures and Breast Cancer Study (WEB Study). *Cancer Epidemiology Biomarkers and Prevention.* 13:1400-1404.

Cruciferous vegetables

Verhoeven, D.T. et al. 1996. Epidemiological studies on brassica vegetables and cancer risk. *Cancer Epidemiology Biomarkers and Prevention.* 5:733-748.

Voorips, L.E. et al. 2000. Vegetable and fruit consumption and lung cancer risk in the Netherlands cohort study on diet and cancer. *Cancer Causes and Control.* 11:101-115.

Deodorants and antiperspirants

Darbre, P.D. et al. 2004. Concentrations of parabens in human breast tumours. *Journal of Applied Toxicology.* 24:5-13.

Dabre, P.D. 2003. Underarm cosmetics and breast cancer. *Journal of Applied Toxicology.* 2:89-95.

Harvey, P.W. and D.J. Everett. 2004. Significance of the detection of esters of p-hydroxybenzoic acid (parabens) in human breast tumors. *Journal of Applied Toxicology.* 24:1-4.

McGrath, K.G. 2003. An earlier age of breast cancer diagnosis related to more frequent use of antiperspirants/deodorants and underarm shaving. *European Journal of Cancer Prevention.* 12:479-485.

Mirick, D.K. et al. 2002. Antiperspirant use and the risk of breast cancer. *Journal of the National Cancer Institute.* 94:1578-1580.

Depression

Kroenke, C. et al. 2005. Depressive Symptoms and Prospective Incidence of Colorectal Cancer in Women. *American Journal of Epidemiology.* 162:839-848.

DES

Hatch, E. et al. 1998. Cancer risk in women exposed to Diethylstilbestrol In utero. *The Journal of the American Medical Association.* 280:630-4.

Strohsmitter, W. et al. 2001. Cancer Risk in Men Exposed in Utero to Diethystilbestrol. *Journal of the National Cancer Institute.* 97:545-551.

Titus-Ernstoff, L. et al. 2001. Long-term cancer risk in women given diethylstilbestrol (DES) during pregnancy. *British Journal of Cancer.* 84:126-133.

Diabetes

Adami, H.O. et al. 1996. Excess risk of primary liver cancer in patients with diabetes mellitus. *Journal of the National Cancer Institute.* 88:1472-1477.

Anderson, K.E. et al. 2001. Diabetes and endometrial cancer in the Iowa women's health study. *Cancer Epidemiology Biomarkers and Prevention.* 10:611-616.

Cerhan, J.R. et al. 1997. Medical history risk factors for non-Hodgkin's lymphoma in older women. *Journal of the National Cancer Institute.* 89:314-318.

Larsson, S., N. Orsini, and A. Wolk. 2005. Diabetes mellitus and risk of colorectal cancer: a meta-analysis. *Journal of the National Cancer Institute.* 97:1679-1687.

Lindblad, P. et al. 1999. The role of diabetes mellitus in the aetiology of renal cell cancer. *Diabetologia.* 42:107-112.

Weiderpass, E. et al. 2002. Reduced risk of prostate cancer among patients with diabetes mellitus. *International Journal of Cancer.* 102:258-261.

Weiderpass, E. et al. 1997. Risk of endometrial and breast cancer in patients with diabetes mellitus. *International Journal of Cancer.* 71:360-363.

Zendehdel, K. et al. 2003. Cancer incidence in patients with type 1 diabetes mellitus: a population-based cohort study in Sweden. *Journal of the National Cancer Institute.* 95:1797-1800.

Dry-cleaning

NIOSH Study of Dry-cleaning workers. National Institute for Occupational Safety and Health. 1996. Accessed 03/29/06 at www.cdc.gov/niosh/pgms/worknotify/Drycleaner/html.

Epstein-Barr virus

Alexander, F. et al. 2000. Risk factors for Hodgkin's disease by Epstein-Barr (EBV) status: prior infection by EBV and other agents. *British Journal of Cancer.* 82:1117-1121.

Bonnet, M. et al. 1999. Detection of Epstein-Barr virus in invasive breast cancers. *Journal of the National Cancer Institute.* 91:1376-1381.

Glaser, S.L. et al. 2005. Exposure to childhood infections and risk of EBV-defined Hodgkin's lymphoma in women. *International Journal of Cancer.* 115:599-605.

Hjalgrim, H. et al. 2003. Characteristics of Hodgkin's lymphoma after infectious mononucleosis. *The New England Journal of Medicine.* 349:1324-1333.

Koriyama, C. et al. 2005. Environmental factors related to Epstein-Barr virus-associated gastric cancer in Japan. *Journal of Experimental and Clinical Cancer Research.* 4:547-553.

Niedobitek, G. et al. 2001. Epstein-Barr Virus Infection and Human Malignancies. *International Journal of Experimental Pathology.* 82:149-170.

Perrigoue, J. et al. 2005. Lack of Association between EBV and breast carcinoma. *Cancer Epidemiology Biomarkers and Prevention.* 14:809-814.

Thompson, M., and R. Kurzock. 2004. Epstein-Barr virus and cancer. *Clinical Cancer Research.* 10: 803-821.

Exercise

American Cancer Society recommendations for nutrition and physical activity for cancer prevention. 2001. Accessed 02/16/06 at www.cancer.org/docroot/PED/content/PED_3_2X_Recommendations.asp?sitearea=PED.

Bernstein, L. et al. 2005. Lifetime recreational exercise activity and breast cancer risk among black women and white women. *Journal of the National Cancer Institute.* 97:1671-1679.

Chao, A. et al. 2004. Amount, type, and timing of recreational physical activity in relation to colon and rectal cancer in older adults: the Cancer Prevention Study II Nutrition Cohort. *Cancer Epidemiology Biomarkers and Prevention.* 13:2187-2195.

Friedenreich, C.M., and M.R. Orenstein. 2002. Physical activity and cancer prevention: etiologic evidence and biological mechanisms. *The Journal of Nutrition.* 132:3456S-3464S.

Governor's Fit School Program. Minnesota Department of Public Health. Accessed 06/05/06 at www.health.state.mn.us/fitschool.

Lagerros, Y., S. Hsieh, and C. Hsieh. 2004. Physical activity in adolescence and young adulthood and breast cancer risk: a quantitative review. *European Journal of Cancer Prevention.* 13:5-12.

Lee, I.M. 2003. Physical activity and cancer prevention—data from epidemiologic studies. *Medicine and Science in Sports and Exercise.* 35:1823-1827.

Michna, L. et al. 2006. Inhibitory effects of voluntary running wheel exercise on UVB-induced skin carcinogenesis in SKH-1 mice. *Carcinogenesis.* Advance Access Published online 05/13/06. Accessed 05/28/06 at http.//carcin.oxfordjournals.org/cgi/search?fulltext=exercise+skin+cancer&x=21%y=12.

Patel, A.V. 2003. Recreational physical activity and risk of postmenopausal breast cancer in a large cohort of US women. *Cancer Causes and Control.* 14:519-529.

Roberts, D.F. et al. 1999. Kids and Media at the New Millennium: A Comprehensive National Analysis of Children's media use. Menlo park, CA: The Henry J. Kaiser Family Foundation Report.

Vincent, S. et al. 2003. Activity Levels and Body Mass Index of Children in the United States, Sweden, and Australia. *Medicine and Science in Sports and Exercise.* 35:1367-1873.

Fast food

Pereira, M. et al. 2005. Fast food, Weight gain, and Insulin Resistance (The CARDIA study): 15 year prospective analysis. *Lancet.* 365:36-42.

Fat types

King, I. et al. 2005. Serum Trans-Fatty Acids are Associated with Risk of Prostate Cancer in B-Carotene and Retinol Efficacy Trial. *Cancer Epidemiology Biomarkers and Prevention.* 14:988-992.

Kobayashi, N. et al. 2006. Effect of Altering Dietary *w*-6/*w*-3 Fatty Acid Ratios on Prostate Cancer Membrane Composition, Cyclooxygenase-2, and Prostaglandin E2. *Clinical Cancer Research.* 12:4662-4670.

Kohlmeier, L. et al. 1997. Adipose tissue trans fatty acids and breast cancer in the European Community Multicenter Study on Antioxidants, Myocardial Infarction and Breast Cancer. *Cancer Epidemiology Biomarkers and Prevention.* 6:705-710.

Questions and Answers about Trans Fat Nutrition Labeling. US Food and Drug Administration. Accessed 04/03/06 at www.cfscan.fda.gov/~dms/qatrans2.html#s1q3.

Velie, E. et al. 2000. Dietary Fat, Fat Subtypes, and Breast Cancer in Postmenopausal Women: a Prospective Cohort Study. *Journal of the National Cancer Institute.* 92:833-839.

Voorips, L. et al. 2002. Intake of conjugated linoleic acid, fat, and other fatty acids in relation to postmenopausal breast cancer: the Netherlands Cohort Study of Diet and Cancer. *Cancer Epidemiology Biomarkers and Prevention.* 76:873-882.

Wolk, A. et al. 1998. A prospective study of Association of Monounsaturated Fat and other types of fat with risk of Breast Cancer. *Archives of Internal Medicine.* 138:41-45.

Fiber intake

Bingham, S.A. et al. 2003. Dietary fibre in food and protection against colorectal cancer in the European prospective investigation into cancer and nutrition (EPIC): an observational study. *Lancet.* 361:1487-1488.

Fuchs, C. et al. 1999. Dietary Fiber Intake and the Risk of Colorectal Cancer and Adenoma in Women. *The New England Journal of Medicine.* 340:169-176.

Park, Y. et al. 2005. Dietary Fiber Intake and Risk of Colorectal Cancer: A Pooled Analysis of Prospective Cohort Studies. *The Journal of the American Medical Association.* 294:2849-2857.

Rohan, T.E. et al. 2002. A cohort study of dietary fibre intake and menarche. *Public Health Nutrition.* 5:353-360.

Fish

Augustsson, K. et al. 2003. A prospective study of intake of fish and marine fatty acids and prostate cancer. *Cancer Epidemiology Biomarkers and Prevention.* 12:64-67.

Fernandex, E. et al. 1999. Fish consumption and cancer risk. *American Journal of Clinical Nutrition.* 70: 85-90.

Fritschi, L. et al. 2004. Dietary Fish Intake and Risk of Leukemia, Multiple Myeloma, and Non-Hodgkin Lymphoma. *Cancer Epidemiology Biomarkers and Prevention.* 13:532-537.

Larssen, S.C. et al. 2004. Dietary long-chain n-3 fatty acids for the prevention of cancer: a review of potential mechanisms. *American Journal of Clinical Nutrition.* 79:935-945.

Norat, T. et al. 2005. Meat, fish, and colorectal cancer risk: the European Prospective Investigation into Cancer and Nutrition. *Journal of the National Cancer Institute.* 97:906-916.

Terry, P. et al. 2001. Fatty fish consumption and risk of prostate cancer. *Lancet.* 357:1764-1766.

Terry, P. et al. 2002. Fatty fish consumption lowers the risk of endometrial cancer: a nationwide case-control study in Sweden. *Cancer Epidemiology Biomarkers and Prevention.* 11:143-145.

Fluid intake

Michaud, D. et al. 1999. Fluid intake and the risk of bladder cancer in men. *The New England Journal of Medicine.* 340:1390-1397.

Negri, E., and C. La Vecchia. 2001. Epidemiology and prevention of bladder cancer. *European Journal of Cancer Prevention.* 10:7-14.

Shanno, J. et al. 1996. Relationship of food groups and water intake to colon cancer risk. *Cancer Epidemiology Biomarkers and Prevention.* 5:495-502.

Stookey, J. et al. 1997. Relationship of Food groups and water intake to colon cancer risk. *Cancer Epidemiology Biomarkers and Prevention.* 6:657-658.

Tang, R. et al. 1999. Physical activity, water intake and risk of colorectal cancer in Taiwan: a hospital-based case-control study. *International Journal of Cancer.* 82:484-489.

Folic acid

Giovannucci, E. 1998. Multivitamin use, folate, and colon cancer in women in the Nurses' Health Study. *Annals of Internal Medicine.* 129:517-524.

Pelucchi, C. et al. 2005. Dietary Folate and Risk of Prostate Cancer in Italy. *Cancer Epidemiology Biomarkers and Prevention.* 14:944-948.

Stolzenberg-Solomon, R.Z. et al. 2006. Folic acid, alcohol use, and postmenopausal breast cancer risk in the Prostate, Lung, Colorectal, and Ovarian Cancer Screening Trial. *American Journal of Clinical Nutrition.* 83:895-904.

Tjonneland, A. et al. 2006. Folate intake, alcohol and risk of breast cancer among postmenopausal women in Denmark. *European Journal of Clinical Nutrition.* 60:280-286.

Free-range chicken and beef/CLA

Aro, A. et al. 1999. Inverse relation between CLA in adipose breast tissue and risk of breast cancer. A case control study in France. *Inform.* 10:5 S43.

Aro, A. et al. 2000. Inverse association between dietary and serum conjugated linoleic acid and risk of breast cancer in postmenopausal women. *Nutrition and Cancer.* 38:151-157.

Fruits

Adams, L.S. et al. 2006. Pomegranate juice, total pomegranate ellagitannins, and punicalagin suppress inflammatory cell signaling in colon cancer cells. *Journal of Agricultural and Food Chemistry.* 54:980-985.

Block, G. et al. 1992. Fruit, vegetables, and cancer prevention: A review of the epidemiological evidence. *Nutrition and Cancer.* 18:1-29.

Bunin, G.R. et al. 2005. Maternal diet during pregnancy and its association with medulloblastoma in children: a children's oncology group study (United States). *Cancer Causes and Control.* 16:877-891.

Jeune, M.S., J. Sumi Diaka, and J. Brown. 2005. Anticancer activities of pomegranate extracts and genistein in human breast cancer cells. *Journal of Medicinal Food.* 8:469-475.

Kwan, M.L. et al. 2004. Food consumption by children and the risk of childhood acute leukemia. *American Journal of Epidemiology.* 160: 1098-1107.

Malik, A. et al. 2005. Pomegranate fruit juice for chemoprevention and chemotherapy of prostate cancer. *Proceedings of the National Academy of Science.* 102:14813-14818.

Maynard, M. et al. 2003. Fruit, vegetables and antioxidants in childhood and risk of adult cancer: Boyd Orr Cohort. *Journal of Epidemiology and Community Health.* 57:218-225.

Pantuck, A.J. et al. 2006. Phase II study of pomegranate juice for men with rising prostate-specific antigen following surgery or radiation for prostate cancer. *Clinical Cancer Research.* 12:4018-4026.

Syed, D.N. et al. 2006. Photochemopreventive effect of pomegranate fruit extract on UVA-mediated activation of cellular pathways in normal human epidermal keratinocytes. *Photochemistry and Photobiology.* 82:398-405.

Garlic

Fleishschauer, A.T. and L. Arab. 2001. Garlic and cancer, a critical review of the epidemiological literature. *The Journal of Nutrition.* 131(3suppl):1032S-1040S.

Mulrow, C. et al. October 2005. Garlic effects on cardiovascular risks and disease, protective effects against cancer, and clinical adverse effects. Agency for Healthcare Research and Quality. Rockville, Md. Evidence report/technology assessment #20. AHRQ publication.

You, W.C. et al. 1989. Allium vegetables and reduced risk of stomach cancer. *Journal of the National Cancer Institute.* 81:162-4.

Gasoline

Hansen, J. 2000. Elevated risk for male breast cancer after occupational exposure to gasoline and vehicular combustion products. *American Journal of Industrial Medicine.* 37:349-357.

Don't Top off your Gas Tank. United States Environmental Protection Agency. Accessed 03/28/06 at www.epa.gov/donttopoff/

Glycemic index

Augustin, L. et al. 2003. Glycemic index and load and risk of upper airo-digestive tract neoplasms. *Cancer Causes and Control.* 14:657-662.

Lagous, M. et al. 2005. Glycemic Load, Glycemic Index, and the risk of Breast Cancer among Mexican women. *Cancer Causes and Control.* 16:1165-1169.

Golf

Kross, B. et al. 1996. Proportionate Morality Study of Golf course Superintendents. *American Journal of Industrial Medicine.* 29:501-506.

Green tea

Baliga, M.S. et al. 2005. Growth inhibitory and antimetastatic effect of green tea polyphenols on metastasis-specific mouse mammary carcinoma 4T1 cells in vitro and in vivo systems. *Clinical Cancer Research.* 11:1918-1927.

Fujimoto, N. et al. 2002. Lung cancer prevention with (-)-epigallocatchin gallate using monitoring by heterogeneous nuclear ribonucleoprotein B1. *International Journal of Oncology.* 6:1233-1239.

Hakim, I.A. et al. 2004. Effect of a 4-month tea intervention on oxidative DNA damage among heavy smokers: role of glutathione s-transferase genotypes. *Cancer Epidemiology Biomarkers and Prevention.* 13:242-249.

Inoue, M. 2001. Regular consumption of green tea and the risk of breast cancer recurrence: follow-up study from the Hospital-based Epidemiologic Research Program at Aichi Cancer Center (HERPACC), Japan. *Cancer Letters.* 167:175-182.

Shanafelt, T.D. et al. 2006. Clinical effects of oral green tea extracts in four patients with low grade B cell malignancies. *Leukemia Research.* 6:707-712.

Sun, C.L. 2002. Urinary tea polyphenols in relation to gastric and esophageal cancers: a prospective study of men in Shanghai, China. *Carcinogenesis.* 23:1497-1503.

Tsubono, Y. et al. 2001. Green tea and the risk of gastric cancer in Japan. *The New England Journal of Medicine.* 344:632-636.

Wu, A.H. et al. 2003. Green tea and risk of Breast Cancer in Asian Americans. *International Journal of Cancer.* 106: 574-9.

Yuan, J.M. et al. 2005. Green tea intake, ACE gene polymorphism and breast cancer risk among Chinese women in Singapore. *Carcinogenesis.* 8:1389-1394.

Zeegers, M.P. et al. 2001. Are coffee, tea, and total fluid consumption associated with bladder cancer risk? Results from the Netherlands Cohort Study. *Cancer Causes and Control.* 12:231-238.

Zhang, M. et al. 2004. Green tea consumption enhances survival of epithelial ovarian cancer. *International Journal of Cancer.* 112:465-469.

Hair dyes

Gago-Dominguez, M. et al. 2003. Permanent hair dyes and bladder cancer: risk modification by cytochrome P4501A2 and N-acetyltransferases 1 and 2. *Carcinogenesis.* 24:483-489.

Takkouche, B., M. Etminan, and A. Montes-Martinez. 2005. Personal use of hair dyes and risk of cancer: a meta-analysis. *The Journal of the American Medical Association.* 293:2516-2525.

Turesky, R. et al. 2003. Identification of Aminobiphenyl derivatives in Commercial Hair Dyes. *Chemical Research in Toxicology.* 16:1162-1173.

Zhang, Y. et al. 2004. Hair-coloring Product use and Risk of Non-Hodgkin's Lymphoma: A Population-based Case-Control Study in Connecticut. *American Journal of Epidemiology.* 159:148-154.

Heavy traffic areas

Knox, E. 2006. Roads, railways, and childhood cancers. *Journal of Epidemiology and Community Health.* 60:136-141.

Hepatitis B

Chang, M.H et al. 1997. Universal Hepatitis B vaccination in Taiwan and the Incidence of Hepatocellular Carcinoma in Children. *The New England Journal of Medicine.* 336:1855-1859.

Van Zonnevold, M. et al. 2004. Long-term follow-up of alpha-interferon treatment of patients with chronic hepatitis B. *Hepatology.* 39:804-810.

Hepatitis C

Duberg, Ann-Sofi et al. 2005. Non-Hodgkin's Lymphoma and other nonhepatic malignancies in Swedish patients with Hepatitis C infection. *Hepatology.* 41: 652-659.

Shiratori, Y. 2005. Antiviral therapy for cirrhotic hepatitis C: association with reduced hepatocellular carcinoma development and improved survival. *Annals of Internal Medicine.* 142:105-114.

Viral Hepatits C. CDC National Center for HIV, STD and TB Prevention. Accessed 05/05/06 at www.cdc.gov/nicdod/diseases/hepatitis/c/faq.htm#7a.

Hormone replacement therapy

Chlebowski, R. et al. 2003. Influence of Estrogen Plus Progestin on Breast Cancer and Mammography in Healthy Postmenopausal Women. The Women's Health Initiative Randomized Trial. *The Journal of the American Medical Association.* 289:3243-3253.

Li, C. et al. 2003. Relationship Between Long Durations and Different Regimens of Hormone Therapy and Risk of Breast Cancer. *The Journal of the American Medical Association.* 289:3259-3263.

Hot foods

Castellsague, X. et al. 2000. Influence of mate drinking, hot beverages and diet on esophageal cancer risk in South America. *International Journal of Cancer.* 88:650-664.

H. pylori

Helicobacter pylori and Peptic Ulcer Disease. Centers for Disease Control and Prevention. Accessed 05/26/06 at www.cdc.gov/ulcermd.htm.

Leodolter, A. et al. 2004. Prevention of Gastric Cancer by Helicobacter pylori Eradication. *Digestive Diseases.* 22:313-319.

Malfertheiner, P. et al. Helicobacter pylori eradication has the potential to prevent gastric cancer: A state-of-the-Art Critique. *The American Journal of Gastroenterology.* 100: 2100-2115.

Simon, J. et al. 2003. Relation of Serum Ascorbic Acid to Helicobacter pylori serology in US adults. The Third National Health and Nutrition Examination Survey. *Journal of the American College of Nutrition.* 22:283-289.

Wong, B.C. et al. 2004. Helicobacter pylori eradication to prevent gastric cancer in a high risk region of China; a randomized control trial. *The Journal of the American Medical Association.* 291:187-194.

Household products

National Institute of Health product database. Accessed 03/26/06 at http://householdproducts.nim.nih.gov/products.htm.

Houseplants

Giese, M. et al. 1994. Detoxification of Formaldehyde by the Spider Plant (*Chlorophytum comoslum* L.) and by soybean (*Glycine max.* L,) cell suspension cultures. *Plant Physiology.* 104:1301-1309.

Wolverton, B.C., W. Douglas, and K. Bounds. 1989. A study of Interior Landscape Plants for Indoor Air Pollution Abatement. *NASA Space Center.*

Wolverton, B.C. *How to Grow Fresh Air: Fifty Houseplants that Purify Your Home or Office.* 1997. New York: Penguin Press.

HPV

Baldwin, S. et al. 2004. Condom use and other factors affecting penile human papillomavirus detection in men attending a sexually transmitted disease clinic. *Sexually Transmitted Diseases.* 31:601-607.

Castellsague, X. et al. 2002. Male circumcision, penile human Papillomavirus infection, and cervical cancer in female partners. *The New England Journal of Medicine.* 346:1105-1112.

Giulano, A. et al. 2003. Dietary Intake and risk of Persistent Human Papillomavirus (HPV) Infection: The Ludwig-McGill HPV Natural History Study. *Journal of Infectious Diseases.* 188:1508-1516.

Harper, D.M. et al. 2006. Sustained efficacy up to 4-5 years of a bivalent L1 virus-like particle like vaccine against human papillomavirus types 16 and 18: follow-up from a randomized control trial. *Lancet.* 367:1247-1255.

Munoz, N. et al. 2002. Role of parity and human papillomavirus in cervical cancer: the IARC multicentric case control study. *Lancet.* 359:1093-1100.

Peto J. et al. 2004. The cervical cancer epidemic that screening has prevented in the UK. *Lancet.* 364:249-256.

Richardson, H. 2005. Modifiable Risk factors associated with clearance of Type-Specific Cervical Human Papillomavirus Infections in a Cohort of University Students. *Cancer Epidemiology Biomarkers and Prevention.* 14:1149-1156.

Scully, C. 2002. Oral squamous cell carcinoma; from an hypothesis about a virus, to concern about possible sexual transmission. *Oral Oncology.* 38:227-34.

Sedjo, R. et al. 2002. Vitamin A, Carotenoids, and risk of persistent Oncogenic Human Paipllomavirus Infection. *Cancer Epidemiology Biomarkers and Prevention.* 11:876-884.

Walboomers, J. et al. 1999. Human Papillomavirus is a necessary cause of invasive cervical cancer worldwide. *Journal of Pathology.* 189:12-19.

Infectious disease

American Cancer Society. Cancers linked to infectious disease. In: *Cancer Facts and Figures.* 2005. Atlanta, Ga. American Cancer Society; 2005

Calattini, S. et al. 2005. Discovery of a new human T-cell lymphotropic virus (HTLV-3) in Central Africa. *Retrovirology.* 2:30.

Infection with Liver flukes. International Agency for Research on Cancer. 1994. Accessed 05/05/06 at www.inchem.org/documents/iarc/vol61/m61-2.html

Klein, E. et al. Identification of a novel retrovirus in prostate tumors of patients homozygous for the R462Q mutation in the HPC1 gene. Presented at the 2006 Prostate Cancer Symposium. Accessed 06/18/06 at www.asca.org.

Lambert, P.F. and B. Sugden. 2004. Viruses and Human Cancer. In: Abeloff MP, Armitage JO, Niederhuber JE, Kastan MB, McKenna WG, eds. *Clinical Oncology 3rd ed.* Philadelphia, Pa: Elsevier Churchill Livingstone. 207-225.

Schistosomiasis. CDC Parasitic Disease Information. Accessed 05/05/06 at www.cdc.gov/ncidod/dpd/parasites/schistosomiasis/factsht_shistosomiasis.htm

Sithithaworn, P. et al. 1994. Parasite associated morbidity: liver fluke infection and bile duct cancer in northeast Thailand. *International Journal of Parasitology.* 6:833-843.

Schottenfeld, D. and J. Beebe-Dimmer. 2006. Chronic Inflammation: A common and Important Factor in the Pathogenesis of Neoplasia. *CA. A Cancer Journal for Clinicians.* 56:69-83.

Wolfe, N.D. et al. 2005. Emergence of unique primate lymphotropic viruses among central African bushmeat hunters. *Proceedings of the National Academy of Science.* 102:7994-7999.

Iron, cholesterol

Lee, Duk-Hee et al. 2005. Heme iron, zinc and upper digestive tract cancer: The Iowa Woman's Health Study. *International Journal of Cancer.* 117; 643-647

Mainous, A. et al. 2005. Iron, Lipids and Risk of Cancer in the Framingham offspring cohort. *American Journal of Epidemiology.* 161: 1115-1122.

Low-fat diet

Beresford, S.A. et al. 2006. Low-fat dietary pattern and risk of colorectal cancer. The Women's Health Initiative Randomized Controlled Dietary Modification Trial. *The Journal of the American Medical Association.* 295:643-654.

Prentice, R.L. et al. 2006. Low-fat dietary pattern and risk of invasive breast cancer: The Women's Health Initiative Randomized Controlled Dietary Modification Trial. *The Journal of the American Medical Association.* 295:629-642.

Lycopene

Agarwal, S. et al. 2000. Tomato lycopene and its role in human health and chronic diseases. *Canadian Medical Association.* 163:739-744.

Bhuvaneswani, V., and S. Nagini. 2005. Lycopene: a review of its potential as an anticancer agent. *Current Medicinal Chemistry Anticancer Agents.* 6:627-635.

Gann, P.H. et al. 1999. Lower prostate cancer risk in men with elevated plasma lycopene levels: results of a prospective analysis. *Cancer Research.* 59:1225-1230.

Hauptmann, M. et al. 2003. Mortality from lymphohematopoietic malignancies among workers in formaldehyde industries. *Journal of the National Cancer Institute.* 9:1615-1623.

Giovannucci, E. et al. 2002. A prospective study of tomato products, lycopene and prostate cancer risk. *Journal of the National Cancer Institute.* 5:391-398.

Giovannucci, E., et al. 1995. Intake of carotenoids and retinol in relation to the risk of prostate cancer. *Journal of the National Cancer Institute.* 23:1767-1776.

Magnetic fields

Ahlbom, A. et al. 2000. A polled analysis of magnetic fields and childhood leukaemia. *British Journal of Cancer.* 83:692-698.

Auvinen, A. et al. 2000. Extremely low frequency Magnetic Fields and Childhood Acute Lymphoblastic Leukemia: An Exploratory Analysis of Alternative Exposure Metrics. *American Journal of Epidemiology.* 151:20-31.

Hatch, E. et al. 1998. Association between Childhood Acute Lymphoblastic Leukemia and Use of Electrical Appliances during Pregnancy and Childhood. *Epidemiology.* 9:234-245.

London, S. 1991. Exposure to Residential Electric and Magnetic Fields and risk of Childhood Leukemia. *American Journal of Epidemiology.* 134:923-937.

Savitz, D. et al. 1998. Case-Control Study of Childhood Cancer and exposure to 60-Hz Magnetic Fields. *American Journal of Epidemiology.* 128:21-38.

Marijuana

Grufferman, S. et al. 1993. Parents' use of cocaine and marijuana and increased risk of rhabdomyosarcoma in their children. *Cancer Causes and Control.* 4:217-224.

Meat, cooking methods, heterocyclic amines

Anderson, K. et al. 2005. Dietary intake of heterocyclic amines and benzo(a)pyrene: associations with pancreatic cancer. *Cancer Epidemiology Biomarkers and Prevention.* 9:2261-2265.

Felton, J. et al. 1994. Effect of microwave pretreatment on heterocyclic aromatic amine mutagens/carcinogens in fried beef patties. *Food Chemical Toxicology.* 32:897-903.

Layton, D. 1995. Cancer risk of heterocyclic amines in cooked foods: An analysis and implications for research. *Carcinogenesis.* 16:39-52.

Tavani, A. et al. 2000. Red meat intake and cancer risk: a study in Italy. *International Journal of Cancer.* 86:425-428.

Ward, M. et al. 1997. Risk of adenocarcinoma of the stomach and esophagus with meat cooking method and doneness preference. *International Journal of Cancer.* 71:14-19.

Medications

Dunnick, J and J. Hailey. 1995. Experimental studies on the long-term effects of methylphenidate hydrochloride. *Toxicology. 103:77-84.*

El-Zein, R. et al. 2005. Cytogenetic effects in children treated with methylphenidate. *Cancer Letters.* 23:284-291.

Rodriques-Manguio, R. et al. 2003. Assessing the economic impact of adverse drug effects. *Pharmacoeconomics.* 21:623-650.

Wysowski, D.K. and L. Swartz. 2005. Adverse drug event surveillance and drug withdrawals in the United States, 1969-2002: the importance of reporting suspected reactions. *Archives of Internal Medicine.* 165:1363-1369.

Medical radiation

Andrieu, N. et al. 2006. Effect of Chest X-rays on the Risk of Breast Cancer Among BRCA ½ Mutation Carriers in the International BRCA ½ Carrier Cohort Study: A Report from the EMBRACE, GENESPO, GEO-HEBON, and IBCCS Collaborators' Group. *Journal of Clinical Oncology.* 24:3361-3366.

Brenner D.J. et al. 2001. Estimated risks of radiation-induced fatal cancer from pediatric CT. *American Journal of Roentgenology.* 176:289-96.

Brenner, D. and C. Elliston. 2004. Estimated Risks Potentially Associated with Full-Body CT Screening. *Radiology.* 232:735-738.

Furtado, C. et al. 2005. Whole-Body CT Screening: Spectrum of Findings and Recommendations in 1192 Patients. *Radiology.* 237:385-394.

Heyes, C.J. and A.J. Mill. 2004. The Neoplastic transformation potential of mammography X-rays and atomic bomb spectrum radiation. *Radiation Research.* 162:120-127.

Pierce, D.A. and D.L. Preston. 2000. Radiation-related cancer risks at low doses among atomic bomb survivors. *Radiation Research.* 154:178-186.

Radiation Risks and Pediatric computed tomography (CT): A Guide for Health Care Providers. National Cancer Institute. Accessed 01/26/06 at www.cancer.gov/cancertopics/causes/radiation-risks-pediatric-CT.

Schwartz, L. et al. 2004. Enthusiasm for Screening in the United States. *The Journal of the American Medical Association.* 291:71-78.

Whole body scanning. United States Food and Drug Administration. Accessed 06/16/06 at www.fda.gov/cdrh/ct/

ACR statement on CT screening exams. American College of Radiology. Accessed 06/16/06 at www.acr.org/s_acr/doc.asp?CID=2192&DID=16014.

Health Risks from Exposure to Low Levels of Ionizing Radiation: BEIR VII-Phase 2. 2005. Accessed 07/21/06 at http://books.nap.edu/catalog/11340.html.

Meditation

Massion, A.O. et al. 1995. Meditation, melatonin and breast/prostate cancer: hypothesis and preliminary data. *Medical Hypotheses.* 44:39-46.

Orme-Johnson, D. 1987. Medical care utilization and the transcendental meditation program. *Psychosomatic Medicine.* 49:493-507.

Schernhammer, E.S. and S.E. Hankinson. 2003. Urinary melatonin levels and breast cancer risk. *Journal of the National Cancer Institute.* 97:1084-1087.

Mediterranean diet

Gallus, S. et al. 2004. Mediterranean diet and cancer risk. *European Journal of Cancer Prevention.* 13:447-452.

Hu, F. 2003. The Mediterranean Diet and Mortality – Olive oil and Beyond. *The New England Journal of Medicine.* 348, 2595-2596.

Knoopes, K.T.B. et al. 2004. Mediterranean diet, lifestyle factors and 10-year mortality in Elderly European Men and Women: The Hale Project. *The Journal of the American Medical Association.* 292:1433-1439.

Trichopoulou, P. et al. 2003. Adherence to a Mediterranean diet and survival in a Greek population. *The New England Journal of Medicine.* 348, 2599-2608.

Melatonin, night-shift workers

Blask, D. et al. 2005. Melatonin-Depleted Blood from Premenopausal Women Exposed to light at night stimulates growth of human breast cancer xenografts in nude rats. *Cancer Research.* 65:11174-11184.

Hansen, J. 2001. Light at night, shiftwork, and breast cancer risk. *Journal of the National Cancer Institute.* 93:1513-1515.

Lie, S.A. et al. 2006. Breast cancer and night work among Norwegian nurses. *Cancer Causes and Control.* 17 39-44.

Massion, A.O. et al. 1995. Meditation, melatonin and breast/prostate cancer: hypothesis and preliminary data. *Medical Hypotheses.* 44:39-46.

Mills, E. et al. 2005. Melatonin in the treatment of cancer: a systematic review of randomized controlled trials and meta-analysis. *Journal of Pineal Research.* 39:360-366.

Rafnssan, V. et al. 2001. Risk of breast cancer in female flight attendants: a population based study. *Cancer Causes and Control.* 12: 95-101.

Microwave heating

Vallejo, F., F.A. Tomas-Barberan and C. Garcia-Viguera. 2003. Phenolic compound contents in edible parts of broccoli inflorescences after domestic cooking. *Journal of the Science of Food and Agriculture.* 83:1511-1516.

Watonabe, F. et al. 1998. Biological Activity of Hydroxo-vitamin B12 Degradation Product Formed during Microwave Heating. *Journal of Agricultural and Food Chemistry.* 46:5177-5180.

Yang, R. et al. 1992. Effects of Microwave radiation on anti-infective factors in human milk. *Pediatrics.* 89:667-669.

Milk

Cho, E. et al. 2004. Dairy Foods, Calcium, and Colorectal Cancer: A Pooled Analysis of 10 Cohort Studies. *Journal of the National Cancer Institute.* 96:1015-1022.

Gao, X. 2005. Prospective Studies of Dairy Products and Calcium intakes and Prostate Cancer Risk: A Meta-Analysis. *Journal of the National Cancer Institute.* 97:1768-1777.

Larsson, S. et al. 2006. Calcium and dairy food intakes are inversely associated with colorectal cancer risk in the Cohort of Swedish Men 1,2,3. *American Journal of Clinical Nutrition.* 83:667-673.

Larsson, S. et al. 2006. Milk, milk products and lactose intake and ovarian cancer risk: A meta-analysis of epidemiological studies. *International Journal of Cancer.* 118:431-441.

Mothballs

Kato, I. et al. 2004. Pesticide Product use and risk of Non-Hodgkin's Lymphoma in Women. *Environmental Health Perspectives.* 112:1275-1281.

Mouthwash

Elmore, J.G. and R.I. Horwitz. 1995. Oral cancer and mouthwash use: evaluation of the epidemiological evidence. *Otolaryngeal Head and Neck Surgery.* 113:253-261.

Multivitamins

Fairfield, K. and R. Fletcher. 2002. Vitamins for Chronic Disease Prevention in Adults. Scientific Review. *The Journal of the American Medical Association.* 287:3116-3126.

Fletcher, R. and K. Fairfield. 2002. Vitamins for Chronic Disease Prevention in Adults. Clinical Applications. *The Journal of the American Medical Association.* 287:3127-3129.

Lichtenstein, A. and R. Russell. 2005. Essential Nutrients: Food or Supplements? Where Should the Emphasis Be? *The Journal of the American Medical Association.* 294:351-358.

Patterson, R.E. et al. 1997. Vitamin supplementation and cancer risk: the epidemiological evidence. *Cancer Causes and Control.* 8:786-802.

Nitrites, hot dogs

Huncharek, M. and B. Kupelnick. 2004. A Meta-Analysis of Maternal Cured Meat Consumption during Pregnancy and the Risk of Childhood Brain Tumors. *Neuroepidemiology.* 23:78-84.

Peters, J.M. et al. 1994. Processed meats and risk of childhood leukemia. *Cancer Causes and Control.* 5:195-202.

Sarasua, S., and D.A. Savitz. 1994. Cured and broiled meat consumption in relation to childhood cancer: Denver. *Cancer Causes and Control.* 5:141-148.

Nuclear facilities

Jablon, S., S. Hrubec and J.D. Boice, Jr. 1991. Cancer in populations living near nuclear facilities. A survey of mortality nationwide and incidence in two studies. *The Journal of the American Medical Association.* 265:1403-1308.

Nutrition

Basiotis, P.P. et al. 2002. The Healthy Eating Index: 1999-2000. Washington, D.C.: U.S. Department of Agriculture, Center for Nutrition Policy and Promotion.

Cline, F. and J. Fay. *Parenting With Love and Logic: Teaching Children Responsibility.* 1990. Colorado: Pinon Press.

Gallop, R. and R. Gallop. *The G.I. Diet. The Healthy, Green-light Way to Manage Weight for Your Entire Family.* 2005. Random House Canada.

Mix It Up. Accessed 07/31/06 at www.mixitupmeals.com.

Munoz, K. et al. 1997. Food Intakes of U.S. Children and Adolescents Compared with Recommendations. *Pediatrics.* 100:323-329.

Seattle Sutton. Accessed 07/31/06 at www.seattlesutton.com.

USDA National nutrient Database for Standard Reference. Release 18. Nutrient Lists. Accessed 3/8/06 at www.ars.usda.gov/Services/docs.htm?docid=9673.

2000 Dietary Guidelines for Americans. Accessed 03/31/06 at www.usda.gov/cnpp/DietGd.pdf.

Wilson, M., M.B. Lagerborg and M. Wilson. *Once-A-Month Cooking,* revised edition. 1999. New York: St. Martin's Press.

Wu, X. et al. 2004. Lipophilic and Hydrophilic Antioxidant Capacities of Common Foods in the United States. *Journal of Agricultural and Food Chemistry.* 52:4026-4037.

Obesity

Bianchini, F. et al. 2002. Overweight, obesity, and Cancer Risk. *Lancet Oncology.* 3:565-574.

Calle, E. et al. 2003. Overweight, Obesity, and Mortality from Cancer in a Prospectively Studied Cohort of U.S. Adults. *The New England Journal of Medicine.* 348:1625-1638.

Flegal, K.M. et al. 2005. Excess Deaths Associated with Underweight, Overweight, and Obesity. *The Journal of the American Medical Association.* 293:1861-1867.

McTiernan, A. 2005. Obesity and Cancer: the risks, science, and potential management strategies. *Oncology.* 7:871-881.

National Health Priorities: Reducing Obesity, Heart Disease, Cancer, Diabetes, and Other Diet- and Inactivity-Related Diseases, Costs and Disability. 2006. National Alliance for Nutrition and Activity (NANA). Accessed 08/04/06 at www.cspinet.org/nutritionpolicy/briefingbook.pdf.

Nielsen, S.J. and B. Popkin. 2003. Patterns and Trends in Food Portion Sizes 1977-1998. *The Journal of the American Medical Association.* 289:450-453.

Ogden, C. et al. 2006. Prevalence of Overweight and Obesity in the United States 1999-2004. *The Journal of the American Medical Association.* 295:1439-1555.

Olshansky, S.T. et al. 2005. A Potential Decline in Life Expectancy in the U.S. in the 21st Century. *The New England Journal of Medicine.* 352:1138-1145.

Shade, E. et al. 2004. Frequent intentional weight loss is associated with lower natural killer cell cytotoxicity in postmenopausal women: possible long-term immune effects. *Journal of the American Dietetic Association.* 104:903-912.

Sinha, R. et al. 2006. Improvement in Risk Factors for Metabolic Syndrome and Insulin Resistance in Overweight Youth who are Treated with Lifestyle Intervention. *Pediatrics.* 117:1111-1118.

Sinha, R. et al. 2002. Prevalence of Impaired Glucose Tolerance among Children and Adolescents with marked obesity. *The New England Journal of Medicine.* 346:802-810.

Vainio, H. and F. Branchini. 2002. IARC handbooks of cancer prevention. Volume 6. *Weight control and Physical Activity.* Lyon, France. IARC Press.

Wonsink, B. and M. Cheney. Super Bowls: Serving Bowl Size and Food Consumption. *The Journal of the American Medical Association.* 293:1727-1728.

Wright, J.D. et al. 2004. Trends in Intake of Energy and Macronutrients – United States, 1971-2000. Center for Disease Control and Prevention's *Morbidity and Mortality Weekly.* 53:80-82.

Occupational exposure

CDC NIOSH Safety and Health Topic: Occupational Cancer. Accessed 02/20/06 at www.cdc.gov/niosh/topics/cancer/.

Hazmap. Occupational Exposure to Hazardous Agents. National Institute of Health. Accessed 06/02/06 at http;//hazmap.nlm.nih.gov/cgi-bin/hazmap_generic?tbl=TblDiseases&id=2.

Hauptmann, M. et al. 2003. Mortality from lymphohematopoietic malignancies among workers in formaldehyde industries. *Journal of the National Cancer Institute.* 9:1615-1623.

Organic foods

Asami, D. et al. 2003. Comparison of the Total Phenolic and Ascorbic Acid Content of Freeze-Dried and Air Dried Marionberry, Strawberry, and Corn Grown using Conventional, Organic, and Sustainable Agricultural Practices. *Journal of Agricultural and Food Chemistry.* 51: 1237-1241.

Brandt, K. and J.P. Molgaard. 2001. Organic Agriculture: Does it enhance or reduce the nutritional value of plant food? *Journal of the Science of Food and Agriculture.* 18:924-931.

Lauridsen, C. et al. 2005. Organic diet enhanced the health of rats. *Danish Research Centre for Organic Farming enews.* Accessed 01/30/06 at www.darcof.dk/research/health.html.

The World of Organic Agriculture. Statistics and Emerging Trends 2006. Accessed 08/07/06 at http://orgprints.org/5161/01/yussefi-2006-overview.pdf.

Willer, Helga and Minou Yussefi. International Federation of Organic Agriculture Movements (IFOAM). The World of Organic Agriculture Statistics and Emerging Trends 2006. Accessed 06/23/06 at www.ifoam.org/

Olive oil

Boyd, G. et al. 2005. Potential anti-cancer effects of virgin olive oil phenols on colorectal carcinogenesis models in vitro. *International Journal of Cancer.* 117:1-7.

Gaynor, M. and J. Hickey. *Dr. Gaynor's Cancer Prevention Program.* New York, NY. Kensington Books, 1999.

LeVecchia, C. and E. Negri. 1997. Fats in seasoning and the relationship to pancreatic cancer. *European Journal of Cancer Prevention.* 6:370-373.

Soler, M. et al. 1998. Diet, alcohol, coffee and pancreatic cancer: final results from an Italian study. *European Journal of Cancer Prevention.* 7:455-460.

Ovarian cancer and green leafy vegetables

Kushi, L.H. et al. 1999. Prospective Study of Diet and Ovarian Cancer. *American Journal of Epidemiology.* 149:21-31.

Pesticides

Buckley, J. et al. 2000. Pesticide exposures in children with non-Hodgkin's lymphoma. *Cancer.* 89:2315-2321.

Burkhart, C. 2004. Relationship of Treatment-Resistant Head Lice to the Safety and Efficacy of Pediculicides. *Mayo Clinic Proceedings.* 79:661-666.

Davis, J. et al. 1993. Family Pesticide use and Brain Cancer. *Archives of Environmental Contamination and Toxicology.* 24:87-92

Fradin, M. and J. Day. 2002. Comparative efficacy of insect repellents against mosquito bites. *The New England Journal of Medicine.* 347:13-18.

Hayes, H. et al. 1991. Case-control study of canine malignant lymphoma: Positive association with dog owner's use of 2,4-Dichlorophenoxyacetic Acid Herbicides. *Journal of the National Cancer Institute.* 83:1226-1231.

Leiss, J. and D. Savitz. 1995. Home pesticide use and childhood cancer: a case-control study. *American Journal of Public Health.* 85:249-252.

Lowengart, R. et al. 1987. Childhood leukemia and parents' occupational and home exposures. *Journal of the National Cancer Institute.* 79:39-46.

Ma, X. et al. 2002. Critical windows of exposure to household pesticides and risk of childhood leukemia. *Environmental Health Perspectives.* 110:955-960.

Menegaux, F. et al. 2006. Household exposure to pesticides and risk of childhood acute leukemia. *Occupational and Environmental Medicine.* 63:131-134.

Pagoda, J. and S. Preston-Martin. 1997. Household pesticides and risk of pediatric brain tumors. *Environmental Health Perspectives.* 105:1214-1224.

Petrochemicals

Yu, Chu-Ling et al. 2006. Residential Exposure to Petrochemicals and the Risk of Leukemia: Using Geographic Information System Tools to Estimate Individual-Level Residential Exposure. *American Journal of Epidemiology.* 164:200-207.

Power lines

Draper, G. et al. 2005. Childhood cancer in relation to distance from high-voltage power lines in England and Wales: A case control study. *British Medical Journal.* 330:1290.

Linet, M. et al. 1997. Residential Exposure to Magnetic fields and Acute Lymphoblastic Leukemia in Children. *The New England Journal of Medicine.* 337:1-8.

Pregnancy, miscarriage, abortion, and cancer

Summary Report: Early Reproductive Events and Breast Cancer Workshop. 2003. The National Cancer Institute. Accessed 01/31/06 at www.cancer.gov/canceringo/ere-workshop-report.

Radon

U.S. Environmental Protection Agency. A Citizen's Guide to Radon: The Guide to Protecting yourself and your family from Radon. 2005. Accessed 01/27/06 at www.epa.gov/iaq/raadon/pubs/citguide.html.

Frequently asked questions about radon. National Safety Council. Accessed 03/28/06 at www.nsc.org/issues/radon/.

Recipes

Grilled Salmon with Teriyaki Shiitake. Dr. Andrew Weil's recipes. February 2006. *Food and Wine.* Accessed 07/27/06 at www.foodandwine.com/recipes/grilled-salmon-with-teriyaki-shitake.

Religious services

Humer, A. et al. 1999. Religious involvement and U.S. mortality. *Demography.* 36:273-285.

Koenig, H.G. et al. 1997. Attendance at Religious Services, Interleukin-6, and other Biological Parameters of Immune Function in Older Adults. *The International Journal of Psychiatry in Medicine.* 27: 233-250.

Oman, D. and D. Reed. 1998. Religion and mortality among the community dwelling elderly. *American Journal of Public Health.* 88:1469-1475.

Oman, D. et al. 2002. Religious attendance and cause of death over 31 years. *International Journal of Psychiatry in Medicine.* 32:69-89.

Sephton, S.E. et al. 2001. Spiritual expression and immune function in women with metastatic breast cancer: an exploratory study. *The Breast Journal.* 7:345-353.

Strawbridge, W.J. et al. 1997. Frequent attendance at religious services and mortality over 28 years. *American Journal of Public Health.* 87:957-961.

Resveratrol

Levi, F. et al. 2005. Resveratrol and breast cancer risk. *European Journal of Cancer Prevention.* 14: 139-142.

Retroviruses, HIV, HTLV-1-4

Calattini, S. et al. Discovery of a new human T-cell lymphotropic virus (HTLV-3) in Central Africa. *Retrovirology.* 2005. 2:30.

Wolfe, N.D. et al. Emergence of unique primate lymphotropic viruses among central African bushmeat hunters. *Proceedings of the National Academy of Science.* 2005. 102:7994-7999.

Salt intake

Buiatti, E. et al. 1990. A case-control study of gastric cancer and diet in Italy; II. Association with nutrients. *International Journal of Cancer.* 45:896-901.

Seaweed

Skibola, C. et al. 2005. Brown Kelp Modulates Endocrine Hormones in Female Sprague-Dawley Rats and in Human Luteinized Granulosa Cells. *Journal of Nutrition.* 135:296-300.

Teas, J. 1983. The dietary intake of Laminaria, a brown seaweed, and breast cancer prevention. *Nutrition and Cancer.* 4:217-222.

Selenium

Combs, G. et al. 1997. Reduction of cancer risk with an oral supplement of selenium. *Biomedical and Enivironmental Sciences.* 3:227-234.

Mark, S. et al. 2000. Prospective Study of serum selenium levels and incident esophageal and gastric cancers. *Journal of the National Cancer Institute.* 92:1753-1763.

Sex

Lee, M.G. et al. 1989. Characteristics of reproductive life and risk of breast cancer in a case-control study of young nulliparous women. *Journal of Clinical Epidemiology.* 42:1227-1233.

Leitzmann, M. et al. 2004. Ejaculation Frequency and Subsequent Risk of Prostate Cancer. *The Journal of the American Medical Association.* 291:1578-1586.

Murrell T.G. et al. 1995. The potential for oxytocin(OT) to prevent breast cancer: a hypothesis. *Breast Cancer Research and Treatment.* 35:225-229.

Petridou, E. et al. 2000. Endocrine correlates of male breast cancer risk: a case-control study in Athens, Greece. *British Journal of Cancer.* 83:1234-1237.

Sleep

Gottlieb, D. et al. 2005. Association of sleep time with Diabetes mellitus and impaired glucose tolerance. *Archives of Internal Medicine.* 165:863-867.

Kliukiene, J. 2001. Risk of breast cancer among Norwegian women with visual impairment. *British Journal of Cancer.* 84:397-399.

Kripke, D. et al. 2002. Mortality Associated with Sleep Duration and Insomnia. *Archives of General Psychiatry.* 59:131-136.

Patel, S.R. et al. 2004. A prospective study of sleep duration and mortality risk in women. *Sleep.* 27: 440-444.

Schernhammer, E.S. et al. 2003. Night-shift work and risk of colorectal cancer in the nurses' health study. *Journal of the National Cancer Institute.* 95:825-828.

Schernhammer, E.S. et al. 2006. Night work and breast cancer. *Epidemiology.* 17:108-111.

Schernhammer, E.S. et al. 2001. Rotating night shifts and risk of breast cancer in women participating in the nurses' health study. *Journal of the National Cancer Institute.* 93:1563-1568.

Reynolds, P. et al. 2002. Cancer incidence in California flight attendants (United States). *Cancer Causes and Control.* 13:317-324.

Tokumaro, O. et al. 2006. Incidence of cancer among female flight attendants: a meta-analysis. *Journal of Travel Medicine.* 13:127-132.

Verkasalo, P.K. et al. 2005. Sleep duration and breast cancer: a prospective cohort study. *Cancer Research.* 65:9595-9600.

Smoking

Clavel, J. et al. 2005. Childhood leukaemia, polymorphisms of metabolism enzyme genes, and interactions with maternal tobacco, coffee, and alcohol consumption during pregnancy. *European Journal of Cancer Prevention.* 14: 531-540.

Johnson, K. 2005. Accumulating evidence on passive and active smoking and breast cancer risk. *International Journal of Cancer.* 117:619-628.

Within 20 Minutes of Quitting. Tobacco Information and Prevention Source. CDC Accessed 05-26-06 at www.cdc.gov/tobacco/sgr/sgr_2004/posters/20mins.htm

Soy

Hirose, K. et al. 2005. Soybean products and reduction of breast cancer risk: a case-control study in Japan. *British Journal of Cancer.* 93:15-22.

Trock, B.J. et al. 2006. Meta-analysis of soy intake and breast cancer risk. *Journal of the National Cancer Institute.* 98:459-471.

Wu, A.H. et al. 2002. Adolescent and adult soy intake and risk of breast cancer in Asian-Americans. *Carcinogenesis.* 9:1491-1496.

Stress

Benson, H. et al. 1974. The Relaxation Response. *Psychiatry.* 37:37-46.

Bernardi, L. et al. 2001. Effect of rosary prayer and yoga mantras on autonomic cardiovascular rhythms: a comparative study. *British Medical Journal.* 323:1446-1449.

Helgesson, O. et al. 2003. Self-reported stress levels predict subsequent breast cancer in a cohort of Swedish women. *European Journal of Cancer Prevention.* 12:377-381.

LeShan, L. *How to Meditate.* New York: Bantam. 1974.

Lutgendorf, S. et al. 2005. Social Support, Psychological Distress, and Natural Killer Cell Activity in Ovarian Cancer. *Journal of Clinical Oncology.* 23:7105-7113.

Saul, A. et al. 2005. Chronic stress and susceptibility to skin cancer. *Journal of the National Cancer Institute.* 97:1960-1967

Sun exposure (see also vitamin D)

Autier, P. et al. 1995. Melanoma and use of sunscreens: an EORTC case-control study in Germany, Belgium and France. *International Journal of Cancer.* 61:749-755.

Autier, P. et al. 1998. Sunscreen use, wearing clothes, and number of nevi in 6 to 7-year-old European children. *Journal of the National Cancer Institute.* 90:1873-1880.

Berwick, M. et al. 2005. Sun exposure and mortality from melanoma. *Journal of the National Cancer Institute.* 97:195-199.

Gallagher, R. et al. 2000. Broad-Spectrum Sunscreen Use and the Development of New Nevi in White Children. *The Journal of the American Medical Association.* 283:2955-2960.

Garland, C.F. et al. 1993 Rising trends in melanoma. An hypothesis concerning sunscreen effectiveness. *Annals of Epidemiology.* 3:103-110.

Grant, W. 2002. An estimate of premature cancer mortality in the U.S. due to inadequate doses of solar ultraviolet-B radiation. *Cancer.* 94:1867-1875.

Green, A. et al. 1999. Daily sunscreen application and betacarotene supplementation in prevention of basal-cell and squamous-cell carcinoma of the skin: a randomized controlled trial. *Lancet.* 354:723-729.

Verne, F. 2003. Preventing Skin Cancer. *British Medical Journal.* 326:114-115.

Westerdahl, J. et al. 1995. Is the use of sunscreens a risk factor for malignant melanoma? *Melanoma Research.* 5:59-65.

Veierod, M.B. et al. 2003. A Prospective Study of Pigmentation, Sun Exposure, and Risk of Cutaneous Malignant Melanoma in Women. *Journal of the National Cancer Institute.* 95:1530-1538.

Supplements

Dietary Supplement Health and Education Act of 1994. United States FDA Center for Food Safety and Applied Nutrition. 12/95. Accessed 06/02/06 at www.cfsan.fda.gov/~dms/dietsupp.html.

Jackson, R.D. et al. 2006. Calcium plus vitamin D supplementation and the risk of fractures. *The New England Journal of Medicine.* 354:669-683.

Nortier, J. et al. Urothelial carcinoma associated with the use of a Chinese herb (Aristolochia fang-chi). *The New England Journal of Medicine.* 342:1686-92.

U.S. Food and Drug Administration. Letter to Health Care Professionals – FDA Concerned About Botanical Products, Including Dietary Supplements Containing Aristolochic Acid. May 31, 2000. Accessed 01/25/60 at www.cfsan.fda.gov/~dms/ds-botl2.html.

Talc

Chang, S. and H.A. Risch. 1997. Perineal talc exposure and risk of ovarian carcinoma. *Cancer.* 79:2396-2401.

Cramer, D.W. et al. 1997. Genital talc exposure and risk of ovarian cancer. *International Journal of Cancer.* 81:351-356.

Gertis, D. 2000. Prospective Study of Talc Use and Ovarian Cancer. *Journal of the National Cancer Institute.* 92: 249-252.

Rosenblatt, K.A. M. Szklo, and N. B. Rosenshein. 1992. Mineral fiber exposure and the development of ovarian cancer. *Gynecologic Oncology.* 45:20-25.

Whittenmore, A.S. et al. 1998. Personal and environmental characteristics related to epithelial ovarian cancer II. Exposures to talcum powder, tobacco, alcohol, and coffee. *American Journal of Epidemiology.* 1128:1228-1240.

Well water

Ayotte, J. et al. 2006. Bladder Cancer Mortality and private well use in New England: an ecological study. *Journal of Epidemiology and Community Health.* 60:168-172.

Chen, Chi-Ling et al. 2004. Ingested Arsenic, cigarette smoking, and Lung Cancer risk: A Follow-up Study in Arseniasis-Endemic Areas in Taiwan. *The Journal of the American Medical Association.* 292:2984-2990.

Chen, K. et al. 2005. The Association between drinking Water Source and Colorectal Cancer Incidence in Jiashan County of China: A Prospective Cohort Study. *The European Journal of Public Health.* 15:652-656.

Kurttio, P. et al. 1999. Arsenic Concentrations in Well Water and Risk of Bladder and Kidney Cancer in Finland. *Environmental Health Perspectives.* 109:705-710.

Vegetables in combination

Campbell, J.K. et al. 2004. Tomato phytochemicals and prostate cancer risk. *Journal of Nutrition.* 134:3486S-3492S.

Canene-Adams, K. et al. 2005. The Tomato as a functional food. *Journal of Nutrition.* 135:1226-1230.

Vitamin A

Hunter, D. et al. 1993. A Prospective Study of the Intake of Vitamins C, E, and A and the Risk of Breast Cancer. *The New England Journal of Medicine.* 329:234-240.

Omenn, G.S. et al. 1996. Effects of a combination of beta caroten and vitamin A on lung cancer and cardiovascular disease. *The New England Journal of Medicine.* 334:1150-1155.

Vitamin B6

Larsson, S. et al. 2005. Vitamin B6 intake, alcohol consumption, and colorectal cancer: a longitudinal population-based cohort of women. *Gastroenterology.* 128:1830-1837.

Vitamin D (see also sun exposure)

Bischoff-Ferrari, H.A. et al. 2006. Estimation of optimal serum concentration of 25-hydroxyvitamin D for multiple health outcomes. *American Journal of Clinical Nutrition.* 84:18-28.

Garland, C. et al. 2006. The Role of Vitamin D in Cancer Prevention. *American Journal of Public Health.* 96:252-261.

Garland, C.F. 2003. More on preventing skin cancer: Sun avoidance will increase incidence of cancers overall. *British Medical Journal.* 327:1228-1228.

Grant, W.B. 2002. An estimate of premature cancer mortality in the U.S. due to inadequate doses of solar ultraviolet-B radiation. *Cancer.* 94:1867-1875.

John, E.M et al. 1992. Vitamin D and breast cancer risk: The NHANES I epidemiologic follow-up study, 1971-1975. *Cancer Epidemiology Biomarkers and Prevention.* 1998. 8:399-406.

Mizoue, T. 2004. Ecological Study of Solar Radiation and Cancer Mortality in Japan. *Health Physics.* 87:532-538.

Schwartz, G. and W. Blot. 2006. Vitamin D Status and Cancer Incidence and Mortality: Something New under the Sun. *Journal of the National Cancer Institute.* 98:451-459.

Vitamin E

Hernandez, L. et al. 2004. Intake of vitamin E (2-R isomers of alpha-tocopherol) and gamma-tocopherol in a case-control study and bladder cancer risk. *Proceeding of the American Association for Cancer Research.* Vol 45. AACR Meeting Abstracts Online. Accessed 07/29/06 at www.aacr.org/.

Wood dust

Barcenas, C. et al. 2005. Wood dust exposure and the association with lung cancer risk. *American Journal of Industrial Medicine.* 47:349-357.

Demers, P.S. and P. Boffeta. 1998. Cancer risk from occupational exposure to wood dust, A pooled analysis of epidemiological studies. *International Agency for Research on Cancer. Technical Report No. 30.* Lyons France.

Wu, X. et al. 1995. A case-control study of wood dust exposure, mutagen sensitivity, and lung cancer risk. *Cancer Epidemiology Biomarkers and Prevention.* 4:583-588.

Wood stoves, fireplaces

Clean Burning Wood Stoves and Fireplaces. Environmental Protection Agency. Accessed 06/01/06 at www.epa.gov/woodstoves.healthier.html

Yoga

Regular yoga practice may help prevent middle age spread. *Science Daily.* 07/21/05. Accessed 04/03/06 at www.sciencedaily.com/releases/2005/07/050720064358.htm.

INDEX

L

M

N

O

P

About the Authors

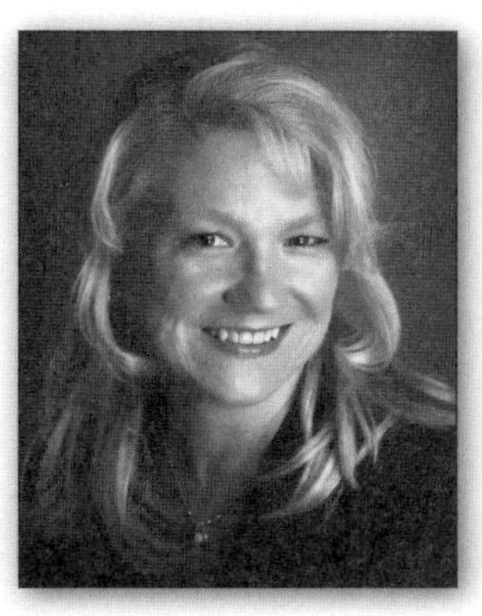

Lynne Eldridge, M.D.

Dr. Eldridge graduated from the University of Minnesota medical school with prestigious Alpha Omega Alpha honors. She completed her residency through the University of Minnesota with time spent in Hawaii studying human exposure to pesticides. Dr. Eldridge passionately practiced family medicine with an emphasis on prevention for over 15 years in Minnesota, before devoting herself full time to researching and speaking internationally on cancer prevention and nutrition.

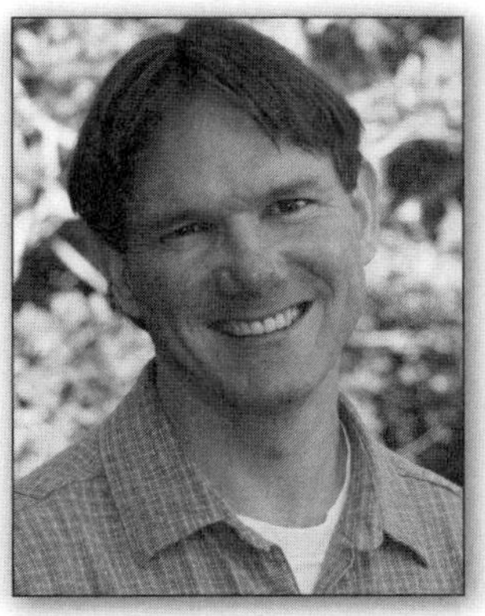

David Borgeson, MS, MPT

David Borgeson graduated with a Master of Science degree in epidemiology from the University of Hawaii and has worked as an epidemiologist and research scientist with the California, Minnesota, and Hawaii State Health Departments. David also holds a Masters degree in Physical Therapy from Northwestern University Medical School, and emphasizes health promotion in his clinical practice. David is Lynne Eldridges brother.

For the latest news in cancer prevention or to contact the authors, check out
www.avoidcancernow.com